T0146262

Understanding Behavioral Health Technicians Within the Military

A Review of Training, Practice, and Professional Development

Stephanie Brooks Holliday, Kimberly A. Hepner, Terri Tanielian, Amanda Meyer, Harold Alan Pincus

Prepared for the Psychological Health Center of Excellence

For more information on this publication, visit www.rand.org/t/RR2649

Library of Congress Cataloging-in-Publication Data is available for this publication.
ISBN: 978-1-9774-0221-9

Published by the RAND Corporation, Santa Monica, Calif.
© Copyright 2019 RAND Corporation
RAND® is a registered trademark.

Support RAND

Make a tax-deductible charitable contribution at
www.rand.org/giving/contribute

www.rand.org

Preface

The military service branches employ a range of health care professionals to meet the diverse health care needs of their beneficiary population. Addressing the behavioral health issues among service members and their families remains a priority for the Military Health System (MHS). Care extenders, part of the health workforce, are members of the care team that provide supportive clinical services alongside licensed independent providers. Behavioral health technicians (BHTs) are enlisted service members who complete technical training to serve as care extenders to licensed mental health providers. BHTs are a key part of the behavioral health workforce. Although BHTs receive substantial training to perform a range of clinical activities, including triage, assessment, counseling, and prevention, to date there has not been a full assessment of the extent to which their selection, preparation, training, and assessment matches the breadth of their roles (in terms of the roles and functions they have been anticipated to play and those that they have undertaken in the field). Accordingly, in recent years, the MHS has demonstrated an interest in better understanding the training of BHTs and the clinical roles that they fulfill.

The Psychological Health Center of Excellence (PHCoE) asked the RAND National Defense Research Institute to assess the current functional operation and utilization of BHTs within the MHS and develop actionable recommendations for optimizing the engagement of BHTs in the MHS. This includes understanding how BHTs function in different military health contexts and identifying optimal roles and needed training and preparation to fulfill these roles. This project has two components. The first component includes a review of the relevant curriculum, policies, and literature, which aims to document the training, roles, and scope of practice of BHTs across the military branches. The second component, to occur at a later time and not addressed in this report, includes a survey of BHTs and licensed mental health providers, with the goal of understanding BHT and provider perceptions of BHTs, their involvement in various clinical activities both in garrison and while deployed, and how BHTs could be used more effectively. This report presents the results of the first component of this study, documenting the results of the curriculum, policy, and literature review.

This research was sponsored by PHCoE and conducted within the Forces and Resources Policy Center of the RAND National Defense Research Institute, a federally funded research and development center sponsored by the Office of the Secretary of Defense, the Joint Staff, the Unified Combatant Commands, the Navy, the Marine Corps, the defense agencies, and the defense Intelligence Community.

For more information on the RAND Forces and Resources Policy Center, see www.rand.org/nsrd/ndri/centers/frp or contact the director (contact information is provided on the webpage).

Contents

Figures and Tables

Figures

Tables

Summary

A top priority for the Military Health System (MHS) is to ensure the efficiency and effectiveness of behavioral health care. An important aspect of this priority is employing an adequate number of mental health providers to meet the needs of service members and their families. Behavioral health technicians (BHTs) are an important part of the MHS mental health care workforce, along with licensed providers, such as psychiatrists, psychiatric nurse practitioners, psychologists, and social workers. BHTs are enlisted service members who receive technical training to support licensed providers and help increase the reach of mental health care within the MHS. However, there can be substantial variability in the ways that BHTs are used across clinical settings, making it difficult to verify that the MHS is making the best use of BHTs' skills.

There has been considerable interest in this use of care extenders (i.e., members of the care team who provide supportive clinical services alongside licensed independent providers) in the military behavioral health context. In 2017, the Psychological Health Center of Excellence formed the Behavioral Health Technician Work Group, which brings together BHTs, mental health providers, and other key stakeholders to evaluate the preparation and use of BHTs and to develop recommendations for how BHTs may be used more effectively to improve quality of care (Blair and Kelley, 2017). And the National Defense Authorization Act for Fiscal Year 2017 mandated a study of mental health care extenders, such as BHTs, to explore their role in increasing access to mental health care for service members and their families (Pub. L. 114-328, 2016). To inform these initiatives, the Psychological Health Center of Excellence asked the RAND Corporation to assess the current functional operation and utilization of BHTs within the MHS and to develop actionable recommendations for optimizing the engagement of BHTs.

To learn more about the training that BHTs receive, we reviewed various curriculum materials, conducted a site visit, and spoke with individuals familiar with BHT training and professional development. To better understand how they are employed in the workforce, we also reviewed service-specific and MHS policies related to the role, scope of practice, supervisory expectations, and competency assessment of BHTs. We supplemented this review with discussions with licensed providers and BHT representatives from each service branch, including program administrators, instructors, and students, who provided context for the policies we reviewed and helped us identify additional relevant documents. We also conducted a literature review focused on the role of military BHTs, which revealed a limited amount of peer-reviewed literature on military BHTs, the majority of which focused on the role of BHTs as part of larger behavioral health teams. There is some overlap in the roles and responsibilities of military BHTs and civilian psychiatric technicians and mental health care extenders. Therefore, we found it helpful to supplement our review of the BHT-focused literature with a search of research on care extenders in civilian behavioral health settings. We also conducted a search related to care extenders in civilian medical contexts to identify best practices for training, practice, and professional development.

Collectively, these sources revealed that BHTs receive a broad educational foundation and training that is applicable to a range of settings, but it remains unclear whether and to what extent BHTs are prepared to fulfill the roles expected of them, especially in deployed or operational settings. There also appears to be inconsistency in how BHTs are utilized across the MHS; in some cases, installations may not be leveraging the full extent of BHTs' clinical training. Additional research could clarify the reasons for these inconsistencies.

This report provides a preliminary foundation for identifying barriers to optimizing the role of BHTs and potential solutions to address these barriers. In follow-on work, RAND will survey BHTs and licensed mental health providers who work within the MHS to collect additional insights on how BHTs are used in practice, their preparedness for fulfilling these roles, and the barriers that may prevent them from being used most effectively.

BHT Selection and Training Vary by Service Branch

The selection process to enter the BHT career field differs by service branch. Figure S.1 provides an overview of the entry requirements for BHTs in the Army, Air Force, and Navy. As of 2016, the latest year for which we had data, 515 students were expected to begin training to become a BHT; of those, 314 were from the Army, 157 were from the Air Force, and 44 were from the Navy (Air Education and Training Command, 2015).

Navy BHT candidates are selected from a pool of personnel who have already been trained as hospital corpsmen. In addition, the Navy's BHT screening process includes a medical evaluation by a psychiatrist, psychologist, or medical officer; candidates are generally not eligible if they have a history of substance abuse, as described in the *Catalog of Navy Training Courses* (CANTRAC) (U.S. Navy, undated).

Army candidates enter specialized BHT training directly from basic training. BHT candidates are accepted for training if they meet or exceed a set minimum score on the Skilled Technical component of the Armed Services Vocational Aptitude Battery (U.S. Army, 2013a), in addition to meeting other qualifications. Air Force enlisted service members also enter BHT training directly from basic military training. Air Force selection criteria include an interview with a mental health provider and completion of a psychological assessment.

In 2010, the three services agreed to use a consolidated training program with a standardized curriculum at the Medical Education and Training Campus (METC) at Fort Sam Houston in San Antonio, Texas. This training focuses on such topics as psychopathology, clinical assessment, and intervention skills and includes both coursework and practicum training at one of ten sites in the San Antonio area (Medical Education and Training Campus, 2018a).

After BHT candidates complete this consolidated program, they receive service-specific coursework and practicum training. In the Army and Air Force, this includes a joint program of medical coursework; Navy BHT candidates complete this basic medical instruction prior to selection as part of their corpsmen training.

Each service relies on unique selection and screening processes. Each has certain strengths; for example, the Air Force requirements are likely designed to ensure that candidates are suitable from a mental health and personality perspective. But although these measures are an important first step in determining suitability for the career field, these procedures do not assess skills or characteristics that are more specific to the BHT career—for example, comfort with one-on-one contact with others, interpersonal sensitivity, or ability to demonstrate empathy. Therefore, there is a need to further assess whether current selection processes adequately identify BHT candidates whose skills, interests, and personality attributes are a fit for the job, which requires substantial face-to-face contact with individuals who are experiencing potentially sensitive issues.

In addition, the breadth and pace of the curriculum in relation to the number of hours of instruction and hands-on practice make it challenging to cover topics essential to clinical practice (as determined through a review of foundational documents and expected competencies from each service branch) in much detail. Training occurs in 14 to 17 weeks, depending on the service, at which point BHTs are expected to enter the workforce, leaving them limited opportunity for future training. This condensed training schedule offers little chance to actually practice the breadth of clinical skills BHTs are expected to learn. Moreover, the Introduction to Counseling course provides a brief overview of many types of theoretical orientations, but it is unclear to what extent the counseling techniques that are taught are derived from evidence-based psychotherapies, though counseling is an expected role of BHTs in some clinical settings. Students also receive few templates or tools to assist in structuring these interactions (Headquarters, Department of the Army, 2017b; U.S. Air Force, 2017). Also, while some courses are designed to provide a broad overview of many topics (e.g., the Psychopathology course covers all DSM diagnoses, including those that are seen infrequently in clinical settings), it means they may not receive in-depth instruction on the diagnoses or clinical techniques most common in the military practice settings in which they will be working (e.g., opportunities to practice the application of this instruction, which is consistent with best practices in training of mental health personnel [Beidas and Kendall, 2010]).

Finally, although the METC is authorized for Army, Air Force, and Navy instructors on the basis of projected student throughput, there are instructor shortages (e.g., the Army fills 80 percent of its positions). As a result, instructors may be overextended, and students may have little opportunity to observe "ideal" intakes or counseling sessions—for instance, as demonstrated by two instructors—prior to attempting the skill themselves under instructor observation or in clinical settings under supervision, as the use of these activities is at the discretion of the instructor.

Moreover, we found that these challenges persist after BHTs begin working in the MHS, with limited guidance on the expectations or requirements for supervision, ongoing training, and professional development of BHTs.

There Is Inconsistency in BHT Roles and Responsibilities

After completing their training at the METC, BHTs become part of the MHS behavioral health workforce. For example, they may be assigned to an outpatient or inpatient clinic at a military treatment facility (MTF) or embedded with a deployed behavioral health team. Once they enter the workforce, BHTs are expected to perform a wide range of clinical tasks, including screening and assessment, intervention, case management, and outreach and prevention. In deployed or operational settings, their responsibilities may be more expansive. However, the literature and our key informant discussions suggested that other responsibilities may take away from time spent on clinical duties, such as administrative responsibilities (e.g., answering phones), facility-level tasks (e.g., serving as inspection control monitors), and unit responsibilities (e.g., motor pool) (U.S. Department of Defense Task Force on Mental Health, 2007; Hoyt, 2017; Nielson, 2016). In turn, the time spent in clinical versus other activities can have important implications for deployment readiness, as BHTs may have little experience with the tasks they are expected to perform while deployed.

There are other key challenges. First, BHTs require on-the-job training (OJT) to develop these skills, but there appears to be no standard expectation as to how to operationalize OJT, ensure that it builds in a meaningful way on the METC training, and disseminate and implement it in an effective and standardized manner. Though some services have specific task qualifications (U.S. Department of the Air Force, 2015) or annual competency assessments for BHTs (Headquarters, Department of the Army, 2017a), there may still be variability in how these expectations are operationalized across service branches. In addition, in our discussions, we learned that some BHTs are able to attend professional development training and that some clinical sites have developed their own training programs for BHTs, but these practices are not standard across MTFs or across the services. This means that there can be variability in BHT skills, especially as BHTs are further from their METC training, which heightens concerns about deployment readiness. Some MTFs have developed training curricula for their BHTs in an effort to build upon skills learned at the METC that are based on specific clinic needs; though these curricula likely facilitate the integration of BHTs into clinical tasks, there are no standardized efforts of this nature.

In addition, because BHTs are not credentialed providers, they work under the supervision of licensed mental health care providers.[1] These supervisors are typically a psychiatrist, clinical psychologist, licensed clinical social worker, or advanced practice psychiatric nurse. Depending on where BHTs are assigned, they could have a single, primary supervisor or multiple supervisors. This could translate to significant variation in the roles that BHTs play within their organizations and the responsibilities they are tasked with across the MHS. Moreover, our document review suggested no standard requirements regarding frequency or intensity of supervision, meaning that some BHTs may receive less supervision than is ideal. Though some variability in the degree of supervision may be appropriate, depending on the specific responsibilities of a BHT in a given setting, this also means that development of BHT skills may be inconsistent, which means that BHTs may be unprepared to fulfill the responsibilities expected of them in subsequent assignments.

Given these challenges, and to ensure that BHTs have a more consistent set of clinical skills and are ready to be assigned to deployed roles, there is a need to better understand how such factors as setting, supervisor preferences, and clinic administrative demands affect their roles. There is also a need to identify ways to better standardize the ongoing training and skill set of BHTs to ensure they are prepared to fulfill the roles for which they were trained.

---

[1]   Air Force BHTs complete requirements for credentialing as Certified Alcohol and Drug Counselors (CADCs) and can perform some tasks independently as allowed by clinic program managers.

Figure S.1
Summary of BHT Qualifications, Training, and Placement

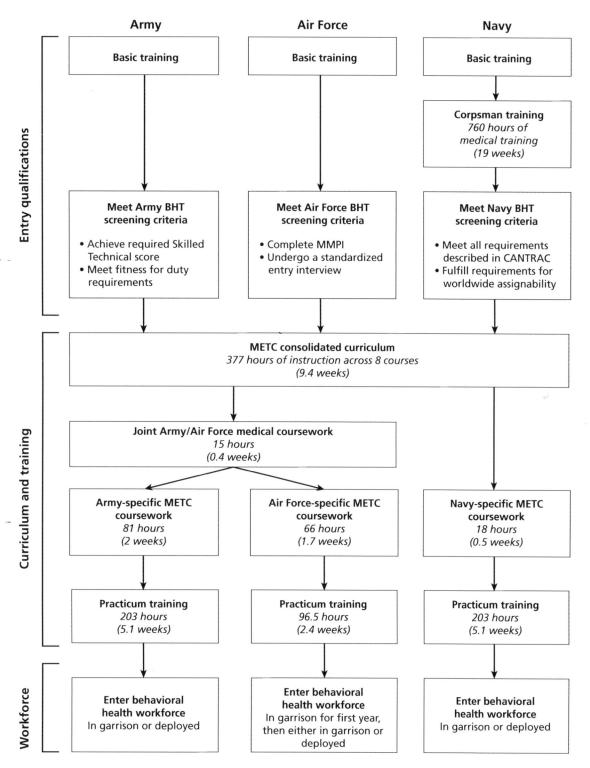

NOTE: MMPI = Minnesota Multiphasic Personality Inventory.

Recommendations

Our review of the selection, training, and professional roles of BHTs pointed to a number of challenges to making the best use of BHTs' clinical skills and promoting the development of these skills throughout their training and after they join the MHS mental health care provider workforce, as summarized in Table S.1.

To address these challenges, we offer the following recommendations.

Recommendation 1. Establish a Consistent Set of Selection Criteria and Candidate Assessment Processes to Ensure Fit with the Career Field

Currently, each service branch uses somewhat different selection criteria. While these differences may be appropriate, as they reflect the priorities and expectations for BHTs in a given branch of service, it would likely be beneficial to establish some minimum standard that reflects the core expectations for BHTs across service branches, especially as health care services become integrated under the Defense Health Agency. For example, the Air Force requires an entry interview prior to entering BHT training. It may be possible to build on this practice and develop a structured entry interview template that all the services could use. Such a template could also assess interpersonal skills to identify a baseline for each candidate and help target instruction in these currently untracked areas.

Table S.1
Summary of Key Challenges to the Effective Training and Use of BHTs

Domain	Key Challenge
Selection	• Selection processes risk selecting BHTs that may lack fit with the job.
Training	• The volume of material covered in the curriculum makes it challenging to cover topics essential to clinical practice in much detail. • Integration of interactive and applied exercises to teach course material can be variable across instructors.
BHT roles and responsibilities in garrison	• BHTs require OJT to develop their skills, but there appears to be no standard expectation as to how OJT should be specifically operationalized, build in a meaningful way on the METC training, and be widely disseminated and implemented in an effective and standardized manner. • BHTs are not consistently used to the full extent of their clinical training, and there is a need to better understand how factors such as the setting, supervisor preferences, and clinic administrative demands affect their roles to determine how they can be used more effectively.
Deployed and operational settings	• It is unclear whether and to what extent BHTs are prepared to fulfill the roles expected of them, especially in deployed or operational settings.
Supervision, ongoing training, and professional development	• There is limited guidance governing specific expectations or requirements for supervision, ongoing training, and professional development of BHTs.

Recommendation 2. Align the Curriculum with Demands of BHTs in the Field and with the Needs of the Population They Serve

Recommendation 2a. Focus the Curriculum on the Conditions That BHTs Encounter Most Often

At the METC, the curriculum is set in alignment with the core competencies expected of BHTs in each service, ensuring that the curriculum covers topics relevant to these competencies. That said, there may be opportunities to better align the curriculum with the roles BHTs play in the field and tailor the curriculum to the populations they serve. This and other adjustments to the curriculum could free up additional instruction hours and provide an opportunity to focus on the most in-demand competencies.

Recommendation 2b. Create Standardized Training Tools That Will Translate to Practice

Although students receive guides for each of their courses, there may be additional opportunities to incorporate standardized tools for training, such as structured intake assessment templates. This would serve as a learning tool at the METC (e.g., by having instructors demonstrate the use of a template and then having students practice using the template) and ensure that all BHTs learn to collect the most important information from patients during clinical encounters.

Recommendation 2c. Teach a Core Set of Evidence-Based Interventions That Generalize to Many Clinical Settings or Patient Populations

During training, the BHT curriculum addresses many psychotherapy techniques, but the counseling techniques students learn to implement are not necessarily anchored in evidence-based psychotherapies. One strategy to bridge the gap between classroom and practice might be to focus the counseling component of the curriculum on a subset of specific, evidence-based, solution-focused interventions that can be implemented across multiple conditions likely to be encountered in the patient populations BHTs will be serving.

Recommendation 3. Standardize Expectations for Involvement in Clinical Activities and Ongoing Training, Clinical Supervision, and Professional Development in the Field

Recommendation 3a. Establish Training Plans for BHTs Entering New Clinical Settings

In our discussions, we learned that some MTFs have made efforts to develop training curricula for BHTs that build on their training at the METC; however, these efforts are not systematic or standard across clinical settings. These types of extended training programs are sometimes used in civilian contexts to improve the integration of care extenders into clinical settings. There may be challenges to implementing one of these typically intensive programs in a military setting (e.g., time required to design training materials, staffing within a given clinic), though less intensive versions of this type of experience could be adapted (e.g., a six- to 12-week training experience at the beginning of each new placement). In turn, there could be benefits to site-specific training to hone newly assigned BHTs' clinical skills. In particular, it would likely facilitate the integration of BHTs into clinical tasks; licensed mental health providers would have more confidence regarding the baseline level of skill of their BHTs, thus ensuring that BHTs are maximally effective as care extenders.

Recommendation 3b. Develop Requirements for Specific Clinical and Educational Experiences

BHTs require substantial OJT and clinical experience to build on the foundational skills they acquire at the METC; however, their involvement in clinical activities may be limited by other responsibilities (e.g., administrative needs), and their clinical experiences can vary greatly depending on the setting in which they are working. If each service identified a core set of skills, centered continuing education requirements around these topics, and clarified expectations and requirements for BHTs, it would help promote readiness and ensure that BHTs maintain baseline skill levels in critical areas. At the moment, it is unclear to what extent BHTs have the opportunity to maintain proficiency in the clinical skills required most commonly in deployed and operational settings, or what those skills may be; however, our survey will provide additional context for expanding on this recommendation.

Recommendation 3c. Establish Requirements or Guidance for Effective Supervision

Our policy review revealed a lack of guidance regarding the necessary or recommended frequency or intensity of supervision. Because BHTs are expected to continue developing the clinical skills they learn during their METC training, supervision is an important consideration. At the moment, it is unclear whether BHTs consistently get necessary feedback or sufficient opportunities for supervision. Our survey will provide additional context regarding the adequacy of supervision; if this does emerge as a common concern of BHTs or licensed providers, implementing policy guidance would help reduce variability in the amount and types of supervision that BHTs receive.

Recommendation 4. Consider Drawing from Best and Innovative Practices in the Civilian Sector for Incorporating Care Extenders into Clinical Care

One challenge that providers and clinics may face is understanding the most effective way to incorporate BHTs so that they truly act as effective clinical team members and complement to licensed provider colleagues, increasing efficiency, access, and quality of care (Schendel, 2018). Here, models and practices commonly used in the civilian sector could hold benefit for clarifying and streamlining the roles and responsibilities of BHTs within the MHS. However, it is possible that the ideal model for better integrating BHTs will depend on the specific setting, workflow, and patient needs.

Limitations

It is important to note the limitations to our findings. First, our review was based on the policy and curriculum documents that were available to us; there are certain documents we may not have been aware of or may not have been able to access. Second, although we conducted key informant discussions, these discussions were conducted with a small number of informants and were focused on providing additional context for the policy and curriculum documents. Finally, though we were able to describe the range of activities that BHTs may engage in, we understand that there is substantial variability in the field.

In this way, this report provides a foundation for understanding the training and roles and responsibilities of BHTs. However, gaps remain in our knowledge, such as the actual degree of variability in tasks conducted in clinical settings, and our review provides limited basis for identifying potential barriers to optimizing the role of BHTs. These are topics that will be covered by our follow-on survey of BHTs and licensed mental health providers, which will provide important data about the ways that BHTs are actually being used in practice, their preparedness for fulfilling these roles, and the barriers that may prevent them from being used most effectively.

Conclusion

Since as far back as World War II, BHTs have been used to increase the capacity of the behavioral health workforce and ensure that service members who need behavioral health care have access to high-quality, efficient services. The demands that BHTs face have undoubtedly evolved alongside the changing needs of the military, but it is unclear whether this valuable component of the MHS mental health care workforce is adequately prepared to fulfill these roles or whether the MHS is making the best use of BHTs' skills. The authors of this report provide preliminary insights on selection, training, roles, and responsibilities. The recommendations presented here will help address variability in these areas and ensure that the MHS can continue meeting the need for high-quality mental health care among service members and their families.

Acknowledgments

We gratefully acknowledge the support of our project sponsor, the Psychological Health Center of Excellence, including TSgt Bradley Blair, MAJ Aimee Ruscio, Peter Kelley, and Dr. Christina Schendel. We appreciate the valuable insights we received from Carrie M. Farmer and Col (retired) Stacey Young-McCaughan, RN. We addressed their constructive critiques as part of RAND's rigorous quality assurance process to improve the quality of this report. We also thank Tiffany Hruby for her assistance in preparation of this report.

Abbreviations

ASVAB	Armed Services Vocational Aptitude Battery
BH	behavioral health
BHOP	Behavioral Health Optimizing Program
BHT	behavioral health technician
CADC	Certified Alcohol and Drug Counselor
CANTRAC	*Catalog of Navy Training Courses*
CBT	cognitive behavioral therapy
CDC	Career Development Course
COSC	Combat Operational Stress Control
DSM-5	*Diagnostic and Statistical Manual of Mental Disorders*, Fifth Edition
FORSCOM	U.S. Army Forces Command
MEDCOM	U.S. Army Medical Command
METC	Medical Education and Training Campus
MHS	Military Health System
MMPI	Minnesota Multiphasic Personality Inventory
MTF	military treatment facility
OJT	on-the-job training
PQS	personnel qualification standards
SOAP	subjective, objective, assessment, plan

CHAPTER ONE

Introduction

Overview

The military service branches employ a range of health care professionals to meet the diverse health care needs of their beneficiary populations. Addressing the behavioral health issues among service members and their families remains a priority for the Military Health System (MHS). To this end, ensuring the appropriate capacity of mental health providers has been a top priority. The mental health workforce within the MHS includes several types of providers, such as psychiatrists, psychiatric nurse practitioners, psychologists, social workers, and behavioral health technicians (BHTs).

BHTs are enlisted service members who complete technical training to serve as care extenders (i.e., members of the care team who provide supportive clinical services alongside licensed independent providers) to licensed mental health providers (Blair and Kelley, 2017). The MHS relies on BHTs as an important part of the mental health work force. BHTs have the potential to increase the efficiency and effectiveness of behavioral health care in the military by providing a core set of clinical services that can streamline clinical operations and increase the availability of licensed mental health providers (Schendel, 2018). In recent years, the MHS has demonstrated an interest in better understanding the training of BHTs and the clinical roles that they fulfill. To this end, in 2017, the Deployment Health Clinical Center (now the Psychological Health Center of Excellence) formed the Behavioral Health Technician Work Group, which brings together BHTs, mental health providers, and other key stakeholders to evaluate the preparation and use of BHTs and develop recommendations as to how BHTs may be used more effectively to improve quality of care (Blair and Kelley, 2017). In addition, the National Defense Authorization Act for Fiscal Year 2017 recently mandated the study of mental health extenders, such as BHTs, to determine how they may increase access to mental health care for service members and their families (Pub. L. 114-328, 2016).

Given this interest in the use of care extenders in the military behavioral health context, the Psychological Health Center of Excellence asked the RAND National Defense Research Institute to assess the current functional operation and utilization of BHTs within the MHS and develop actionable recommendations for optimizing the engagement of BHTs in the MHS. This includes understanding how BHTs function in different military health contexts and identifying optimal roles and needed training and preparation to fulfill these roles. To accomplish this, this project has two components. The first component includes a review of the relevant curriculum, policies, and literature, which aims to document the training, roles, and scope of practice of BHTs across the military branches. The second component, to occur in the future, includes a survey of BHTs and licensed mental health providers, with the goal of understanding BHT and provider perceptions of BHTs, their involvement in various clinical activities both in garrison and while deployed, and how BHTs could be used more effectively. This report presents the results of the first component of this study, documenting the results of the curriculum, policy, and literature review.

The purpose of this report is to (1) describe the selection and training process for BHTs, (2) describe the roles, responsibilities, and ongoing professional development of BHTs, and (3) list key findings and initial recommendations about BHT selection, training, and roles and responsibilities, with the goal of optimizing the role of BHTs in the MHS. In this introductory chapter, we provide an overview of the background and intended use of BHTs and a rationale for examining ways that their roles can be optimized in the MHS.

Behavioral Health Technicians in the Military Health System

Behavioral health care in the MHS is provided in large part by licensed mental health providers, including psychiatrists, psychologists, social workers, and psychiatric nurse practitioners. These clinicians provide care at military treatment facilities (MTFs) and also in embedded roles within units and in deployed settings. BHTs are enlisted service members who complete technical training to serve as care extenders to these licensed mental health providers. Some version of the BHT role has been in place in the MHS from as early as World War II (Harris and Berry, 2013). Since their early days, BHTs have been used to increase the capacity of the behavioral health workforce and ensure that service members in need of behavioral health care have access to high-quality, efficient services. Over the years, the demands on BHTs have evolved as the behavioral health needs of the military have changed. For example, prior to the conflicts in Iraq and Afghanistan, BHTs were designed to provide "basic assessment, counseling and mental health care in both inpatient and outpatient settings under the supervision of licensed providers" (Harris and Berry, 2013). Though these remain the core functions of BHTs today, their training has been updated to reflect behavioral health areas that have become more prevalent (e.g., drug and alcohol treatment, suicide awareness) (Harris and Berry, 2013). Ultimately, the BHT role is designed to provide a range of services in a role that supports mental health providers and increases their ability to serve the military community.

BHTs are trained to fulfill a wide range of clinical needs. Across service branches, these can be largely categorized as screening and assessment (e.g., triage, intake assessments); psychosocial interventions (e.g., brief, solution-focused treatment, psychoeducation); case management (e.g., developing treatment plans); and outreach, prevention, and resilience (e.g., consulting with unit leaders) (Air Education and Training Command Occupational Analysis Division, 2017; U.S. Department of the Air Force, 2015; Headquarters, Department of the Army, 2017b; U.S. Air Force, 2017; U.S. Navy, 2013). However, there are concerns that they are not being used to the full extent of their training, instead being tasked with clerical or administrative roles or pulled for nonclinical military duties. These concerns have been raised by multiple sources: military providers and scholars, a U.S. Department of Defense Task Force on Mental Health, and evaluators of military behavioral health systems of care (U.S. Department of Defense Task Force on Mental Health, 2007; Harris and Berry, 2013; Hoyt, 2017; Srinivasan and DiBenigno, 2016). To better understand the selection, training, and roles and responsibilities of BHTs, we conducted a review of relevant policies, the BHT curriculum, and published literature. In addition to providing important context for this project and the development of the follow-on survey that forms the second component of this study, this review provides an initial opportunity to identify potential recommendations as to how BHTs can be more effectively selected, trained, and leveraged as care extenders in clinical settings.

Curriculum, Policy, and Literature Review Methods

To better understand the education, training, and roles and responsibilities of BHTs, we conducted a review of multiple types of documents and sources. In addition to reviewing the BHT training curriculum and policy documents related to the use of BHTs in the military, we conducted a review of the peer-reviewed literature, including literature specific to military BHTs, as well as literature related to civilian care extenders in behavioral health and other medical contexts. This chapter describes the procedures used to conduct the policy, curriculum, and literature review.[1]

Curriculum and Policy Review

To better understand the nature and content of training received by BHTs prior to entering the career field, we reviewed the BHT curriculum. BHTs from across military services complete their training at the Medical Education and Training Campus (METC) located at Fort Sam Houston in San Antonio, Texas. This training focuses on topics such as psychopathology and clinical assessment and intervention skills and includes didactic and experiential components (METC, 2018a). To better understand the areas in which BHTs receive formal training, we reviewed the curriculum and other relevant documents, including the Course Training Plan (Air Education and Training Command, 2015) and Resource Requirements Analysis Report (Health Care Interservice Training Office, 2015). We also consulted with key informants involved in the training of BHTs (e.g., staff at the METC) to learn more about the curriculum and training cycle and conducted a site visit to better understand the teaching and evaluation techniques used by instructors. During the site visit, we had informal conversations with several key informants, including program administrators, instructors, and students. We also observed students during practical components of their coursework (i.e., practice counseling sessions).

We also conducted a review of policies relevant to the training and practice of BHTs. This included policies focused on the delivery of training at the METC, as well as relevant service-specific and MHS policies related to the role, scope of practice, supervisory expectations, and competency assessment of BHTs. To identify these policies, we reviewed public-facing military websites. We also consulted with members of the BHT Work Group to identify additional policies and other relevant documents.

We supplemented our review of the curriculum and policies with key informant discussions. We conducted eight telephone discussions, which included the representation of at least one licensed provider and one BHT representative from each service branch, which helped us to identify additional policies and provided additional context for the history and implementation of the curriculum and service branch policies. Our discussions also occasionally yielded information about installation-level approaches to ongoing professional development of BHTs,

---

[1]   Note that all procedures were reviewed by the RAND Institutional Review Board and determined to be Not Human Subjects research.

and we reviewed examples of these training curricula developed by providers and/or senior BHTs.

A complete list of the policy and curriculum documents we reviewed appears in Appendix A.

Literature Review

In addition, we conducted a review of the published literature to better describe the role of BHTs in the military. Our literature review had two components. First, we examined literature specific to uniformed BHTs. This element of the literature review was designed to identify information about the training and roles of military BHTs. Second, there is some overlap in the roles and responsibilities of BHTs and civilian psychiatric technicians and mental health care extenders. Therefore, we conducted a review of literature related to civilian care extenders in behavioral health settings (e.g., psychiatric technicians, psychometrists [responsible for administering and scoring psychological tests], mental health care managers), as well as a review of literature related to civilian care extenders in other medical settings. This aspect of the search was designed to provide additional information on the ways that the training and roles of care extenders are structured in other settings and contexts, and to identify any best practices, innovations, or frameworks related to training, clinical roles, or supervision.

Summary

This report provides a description of the selection, training, and roles and responsibilities of behavioral health technicians, as well as key findings and recommendations for each of these stages of the BHT career. In the following chapters, we describe the selection, education, and training of BHTs (Chapter Two), as well as the roles and responsibilities that BHTs fulfill once they enter the workforce (Chapter Three). In each of these chapters, we begin by using the results of the policy and curriculum review, as well as the literature specific to military BHTs to describe the relevant current processes and procedures. This is supplemented, where appropriate, by observations from our site visit to the METC and information from our key informant discussions. We then describe key findings related to selection, education, and roles and responsibilities, with a focus on identifying potential opportunities for improvement or modification to current practices. In these sections, we draw upon the literature focused on civilian behavioral health and medical care extenders to describe innovative and best practices that could be adapted for the military BHT context. Finally, in Chapter Four, we draw on information from across sources to summarize key findings and propose recommendations. Appendix A provides a list of the policy and curriculum documents identified in this review. Appendix B describes the search strategy for each component of the literature search.

CHAPTER TWO

Behavioral Health Technician Selection and Training

Although there are service-specific qualification criteria for the BHT career field, BHTs from across service branches complete a tri-service training curriculum at the METC, on Fort Sam Houston at Joint Base San Antonio (METC, 2018b). In addition to a core curriculum, BHT trainees at the METC also complete service-specific coursework and practical training on campus. In this chapter, we review BHT entry qualifications and describe the education and training that take place at the METC. These descriptions are based on our review of relevant policy and curriculum documents, which were supplemented by key informant discussions and observations made during the site visit to the METC.

Qualifications for Entry into the BHT Career Field

Each service branch has somewhat different requirements for entry into the BHT career field. An overview of training and entry requirements for BHTs across service branches is provided in Figure 2.1.

Training Prior to the METC

In the Army and Air Force, new recruits first complete basic training. There is no additional specialized training prior to entering the BHT program at the METC. Navy BHTs first complete basic training, known as Recruit Training. The next step is to complete the 19-week "A" School, which provides initial education related to patient care (e.g., venipuncture, patient assessment) (U.S. Department of the Navy, 2015; Navy Recruiting Command, 2018; U.S. Navy, 2016). Completion of "A" School qualifies sailors as hospital corpsmen. A subset of these trainees continues on to more specialized training, such as to become a BHT.

Note that the BHT career field is open to service members who may be retraining from another career field.

Eligibility Criteria

Each of the services uses a different process to screen potential BHT candidates. Army service members are eligible if they obtain a score of 101 on the Skilled Technical component of the Armed Services Vocational Aptitude Battery (ASVAB) (U.S. Army, 2013a). Other selection criteria pertain to physical qualifications and absence of criminal justice involvement (e.g., no history of felony conviction or other specific charges) (U.S. Army, 2017a).

Air Force service members must have completed high school or General Educational Development to enter BHT training. In addition, they must complete a Minnesota Multipha-

Figure 2.1
BHT Qualifications for Entry Across Services

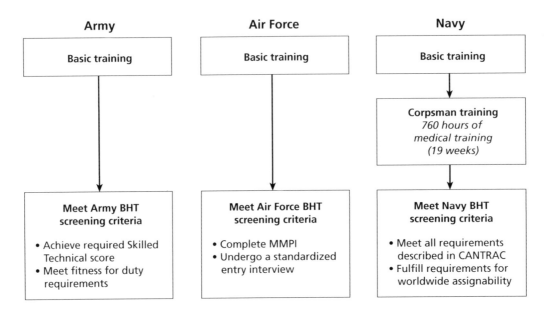

NOTE: MMPI = Minnesota Multiphasic Personality Inventory; CANTRAC = *Catalog of Navy Training Courses.*

sic Personality Inventory-2-Restructured Form (MMPI-2-RF) and "undergo a standardized entry interview," to be completed by a senior BHT or credentialed mental health provider (U.S. Department of the Air Force, 2015; U.S. Air Force, 2017; U.S. Air Force, 2018). However, the nature of the interview and the ways in which the MMPI-2-RF results are used was unclear.

The Navy BHT screening process involves a medical evaluation by a psychiatrist, psychologist, or medical officer; service members are generally not eligible for the position if they have a history of substance abuse, as described in the *Catalog of Navy Training Courses* (CANTRAC) (U.S. Navy, undated). They must also meet all requirements related to worldwide assignability (e.g., no medical conditions that would limit worldwide assignability) (U.S. Department of the Navy, 2012; Health Care Interservice Training Office, 2015).

In 2016, 515 students were anticipated to enter training to become a BHT, including 314 from the Army, 157 from the Air Force, and 44 from the Navy (Air Education and Training Command, 2015). However, we did not have access to information regarding the total number of new enlisted or retraining service members, how many students express interest in entering the career field, and how administrators make decisions regarding filling remaining openings (e.g., are all service members who meet eligibility criteria considered for these remaining openings?). We also did not have information about who in each service is responsible for the selection process for BHTs. This information could be useful in future assessments of how well the services are selecting candidates for the BHT role, though performing that assessment was outside the scope of our study.

BHT Curriculum

Prior to 2010, each of the service branches was individually responsible for the education and training of its BHTs. In 2010, the three services agreed to use a consolidated training program with a standardized curriculum at the METC (Harris and Berry, 2013). The program is accredited by the Community College of the Air Force, and students receive college credits for completion of the course (Air University, 2017). The BHT curriculum at the METC includes three primary elements: (1) a consolidated training component that is completed by students across service branches; (2) service-specific coursework, which covers topics that are specific to the roles played by BHTs in a given service branch; (3) a clinical practicum. In total, from the start of the METC BHT training, Army BHTs complete 676 hours (17 weeks) of training; Air Force BHTs complete 554.5 hours (14 weeks); and Navy BHTs complete 598 hours (15 weeks). Per one key informant discussion, in fiscal year 2018, the Army and Air Force had 12 cohorts that came through the METC, and the Navy had six cohorts.

According to one key informant discussion, the curriculum is set through a review of the foundational documents from each service branch. The goal of this review is to identify the core requirements from each service, and to ensure that these are covered by either the consolidated courses or the service-specific coursework. Generally, the curriculum is reviewed in full each year and every time one of these foundational documents is revised by a service branch. Anytime an update is made to the curriculum based on these reviews, a validation process takes place, which includes teaching the curriculum with all the new materials that were developed, documenting time spent on each objective, surveying students for understanding, and ensuring the accuracy of all materials. It can take three or four cohorts of teaching the new curriculum to complete the validation process.

Each component of the METC curriculum is summarized in Figure 2.2 and described in more detail next.

Consolidated Training

The consolidated training component comprises 377 hours of instruction across eight courses, covered in 9.4 weeks (see Table 2.1). Each of the eight courses includes a didactic component and a written test. In addition, certain courses feature a lab/practical component, which includes demonstration and the opportunity for hands-on practice, as well as a practical test, which is a hands-on student assessment (Clay, 2016). During our site visit, we learned that students receive a student guide for each course, which provides a detailed outline of the material covered. For some courses, there may also be supplemental texts used by instructors.

The initial three courses are didactic in nature, providing an overview of the BHT role and introducing ethical practice (e.g., ethical principles and code of ethics, ethical decision-making), and then moving into biological bases of psychology and theories of development. The final didactic course is Psychopathology, which provides an overview of behavioral health conditions identified in the *Diagnostic and Statistical Manual of Mental Disorders*, Fifth Edition (DSM-5) (Clay, 2016). Given the volume of information covered (e.g., diagnostic criteria for all psychiatric diagnoses), a substantial amount of time is dedicated to this course (85 hours).

After these three didactic courses, the curriculum moves to focus on the clinical skills needed to fulfill the BHT role, including interviewing, psychological testing, and counseling (Clay, 2016). Though each of the next five courses generally begins with a didactic overview of the topic, a substantial amount of time is devoted to hands-on practice. For example, in Inter-

Figure 2.2
BHT METC Curriculum and Training

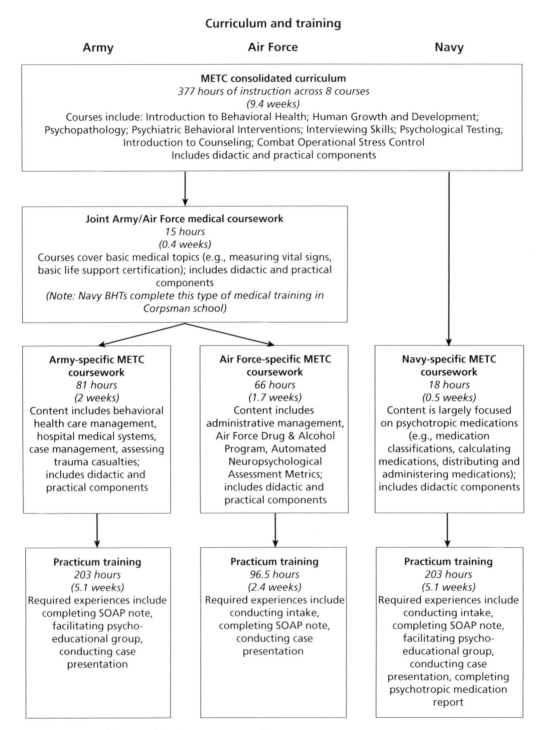

Curriculum and training

Army	Air Force	Navy

METC consolidated curriculum
377 hours of instruction across 8 courses
(9.4 weeks)
Courses include: Introduction to Behavioral Health; Human Growth and Development;
Psychopathology; Psychiatric Behavioral Interventions; Interviewing Skills; Psychological Testing;
Introduction to Counseling; Combat Operational Stress Control
Includes didactic and practical components

Joint Army/Air Force medical coursework
15 hours
(0.4 weeks)
Courses cover basic medical topics (e.g., measuring vital signs,
basic life support certification); includes didactic and practical
components
*(Note: Navy BHTs complete this type of medical training in
Corpsman school)*

Army-specific METC coursework
81 hours
(2 weeks)
Content includes behavioral health care management, hospital medical systems, case management, assessing trauma casualties; includes didactic and practical components

Air Force-specific METC coursework
66 hours
(1.7 weeks)
Content includes administrative management, Air Force Drug & Alcohol Program, Automated Neuropsychological Assessment Metrics; includes didactic and practical components

Navy-specific METC coursework
18 hours
(0.5 weeks)
Content is largely focused on psychotropic medications (e.g., medication classifications, calculating medications, distributing and administering medications); includes didactic components

Practicum training
203 hours
(5.1 weeks)
Required experiences include completing SOAP note, facilitating psycho-educational group, conducting case presentation

Practicum training
96.5 hours
(2.4 weeks)
Required experiences include conducting intake, completing SOAP note, conducting case presentation

Practicum training
203 hours
(5.1 weeks)
Required experiences include conducting intake, completing SOAP note, facilitating psycho-educational group, conducting case presentation, completing psychotropic medication report

NOTE: SOAP = subjective, objective, assessment, plan.

viewing Skills, students learn about the key elements of an intake interview, including a mental status exam and risk assessment. After nearly 20 didactic hours, they spend 38 hours learning to conduct and document an intake interview. In Introduction to Counseling, students

Table 2.1
The METC Consolidated BHT Courses

Course Title	Sample Topics	Format	Total Hours
Introduction to Behavioral Health	BHT duties, ethics	Didactic	10
Human Growth and Development	Anatomy and physiology, human development	Didactic	16
Psychopathology	DSM-5 diagnoses and their signs and symptoms	Didactic	85
Psychiatric Behavioral Interventions	Inpatient procedures, milieu therapy, managing aggressive behavior	Didactic/Practical	37
Interviewing Skills	Mental status exam, risk assessment and management, managing client behavior	Didactic/Practical	88
Psychological Testing	Introduction to psychological tests, including cognitive, personality, and functional assessments	Didactic/Practical	16
Introduction to Counseling	Theoretical orientations, developing counseling goals, group processes, documenting counseling sessions	Didactic/Practical	91
Combat Operational Stress Control (COSC)	COSC across services, crisis intervention, traumatic event management, traumatic brain injury	Didactic/Practical	34

SOURCE: Clay, 2016.

begin by learning about theoretical orientations to counseling, specific therapeutic approaches, and key elements of individual and group counseling. Then, they learn to conduct an individual counseling session, which includes 21 hours spent on the lab/practical component and 21 hours spent on the performance evaluation (Clay, 2016). The final course covers Combat Operational Stress Control (COSC), including teaching students about COSC across the service branches, reviewing crisis intervention and traumatic event management, and a brief practical element performing a combat stress intervention.

The instructor-to-student ratio in these courses is intended to be capped at 1:27 (Health Care Interservice Training Office, 2015). This is designed to ensure that instructors can incorporate small-group activities and interactive exercises. These include activities that would allow instructors to demonstrate the application of course material, such as case studies, videos, and two-instructor role-play demonstrations. For practical exercises, the instructor-to-student ratio is intended to be 1:6, with the goal of ensuring that instructors can spend a substantial amount of time interacting with students to develop these skills (Health Care Interservice Training Office, 2015). To promote this applied practice, the METC is equipped with nine paired observation and counseling rooms, in which the observation room and counseling room are separated by a two-way mirror, and two-way voice communication is possible via intercom (Health Care Interservice Training Office, 2015). During our site visit, we observed these rooms in use for practical components of the intake and counseling courses. Instructors noted that structured scoring rubrics are used to evaluate students during these practical components.

Service-Specific Coursework

Following the consolidated coursework, BHT trainees complete service-specific courses that cover BHT responsibilities that are not common across service branches (Clay, 2016). The Army and Air Force have 15 hours of shared coursework, which covers basic medical topics, including basic life support and measuring vital signs. Because Navy BHTs complete hospital corpsman training before their BHT training, they have already covered this content in more detail.

The remainder of the service-specific coursework is tailored to the role that BHTs play in each respective branch of service (Clay, 2016). Although we did not have access to the student guides for these courses, the curriculum plan provides some broad insight into the nature of these courses. The Army has 81 hours of Army-specific coursework, which provides didactic education in areas such as seizure management, hospital medical systems/programs, and case management. There are also practical components, including learning to conduct a psychoeducational brief and assess trauma casualties. The Air Force requires 66 hours of additional coursework, with didactic elements that cover the role of BHTs in the Air Force Medical Service and administrative management. Additional topics include an overview of inpatient/outpatient services, the Air Force Alcohol and Drug Abuse Prevention and Treatment Program, the Family Advocacy Program, and an introduction to the Automated Neuropsychological Assessment Metrics. The Navy requires 18 hours of additional training, which focuses largely on psychopharmacology.

Service-Specific Practicum Training

The final component of BHT training is a directed clinical practicum (Health Care Interservice Training Office, 2015). The clinical practicum is designed to provide students with the opportunity to practice skills learned during coursework in a clinical setting. There are 10 practicum sites in the San Antonio region, which include military sites and civilian sites (e.g., state hospital, forensic hospital, homeless shelter) with which the military has a memorandum of understanding. These sites provide a mix of inpatient and outpatient experiences, with some also providing exposure to emergency rooms and psychological testing clinics.

Each service branch has slightly different requirements for this element of the training (Clay, 2016). The Army requires 203 hours of practicum training (approximately five weeks). Key elements of this experience include learning to establish therapeutic rapport; documenting subjective, objective, assessment, plan (SOAP) notes; and facilitating a psychoeducational group. The practicum culminates in the preparation and presentation of a case from the practicum site. The Air Force implemented its practicum requirement more recently, in 2015, and currently requires 96.5 hours (approximately two weeks). To maximize clinical experience, Air Force students generally spend about one week at each of two sites. During this practicum, they learn to establish rapport, conduct an intake interview, complete a SOAP note, and prepare and conduct a case presentation. Finally, the Navy requires 203 hours of practicum training (approximately five weeks). In addition to learning to establish rapport, completing a SOAP note, facilitating a psychoeducational group, and conducting a case presentation, Navy BHTs are required to conduct an intake interview, complete a psychotropic presentation report, and learn to triage psychiatric patients.

All supervision for clinical experiences at these sites is provided by the METC instructors. The Army aims for a supervisor-to-trainee ratio of 1:5, while the Navy and Air Force aim for a 1:3 ratio; however, given staffing challenges, the ratio is generally 1:6, which still meets the standards outlined in memoranda of understanding (Health Care Interservice Training Office, 2015).

In the most recent Resource Requirements Analysis, challenges to providing these practicum experiences were reviewed (Health Care Interservice Training Office, 2015). Though starting dates are staggered, multiple cohorts are in training at the same time. Some of the practicum facilities are spread out across the San Antonio area, or place students in multiple locations. This can be a challenge for instructors providing supervision, as students do not have consistent access to their instructors. Staffing becomes a particular challenge during performance tasks. As described previously, each service has a certain number of performance tasks required during the practicum experience (e.g., completing an intake, facilitating a psychoeducational group), which are more instructor-intensive.

Evaluation of Student Performance

In each course and as part of their practicum experience, BHT students complete a written and/or practical test (Clay, 2016). According to one key informant discussion, students are required to pass every exam with a 70-percent or greater score. If students fail three initial exams, or fail the same exam twice, they have to meet an Academic Oversight Board. This Board reviews the student's grades and qualifications (e.g., ASVAB scores) and meets directly with the student about his or her performance. Pending the results of the review, the Board will make a recommendation, such as having the student repeat the training with a new training cohort or reclassifying the student to a different career field. The Dean of Academics makes the final determination as to action to be taken.

Instructor Training and Roles

As of 2015, the METC was authorized for 31 instructors for the BHT course, including 19 Army instructors, eight Air Force instructors, and four Navy instructors (Air Education and Training Command, 2015). These authorizations are based on the projected student throughput. That said, these positions are not always filled (Health Care Interservice Training Office, 2015). For example, the Army staffs the program at 80 percent. This can present a challenge, as instructors may be teaching four courses simultaneously (Health Care Interservice Training Office, 2015). It also presents a challenge for adequately staffing the instructor-intensive directed clinical practicum, as described earlier (Health Care Interservice Training Office, 2015).

Instructors include a mix of officers and senior BHTs (Air Education and Training Command, 2015). According to the BHT Course Training Plan, an officer at the rank of major is required to provide oversight for training, and this individual must be licensed to practice psychology (Air Education and Training Command, 2015). Enlisted instructors must be trained as BHTs and at a grade of E5 or higher. Instructors receive training prior to assuming the position, including an approved instructor methodology course, the METC orientation, and instructor competency development training (Clay, 2016; Navy Medicine, 2018). Instructors must also complete a "12 semester hour teaching internship course, be current in subject matter testing, have satisfactory annual instructor evaluations, and obtain at least one hour of professional development, documented annually" (Clay, 2016, p. 5). Army instructors are also required to attend a Cadre Training Course, which focuses on equipping instructors to work with Initial Entry Training soldiers (i.e., new recruits) (Clay, 2016; Headquarters, Department of the Army, 2017c).

Key Challenges in BHT Selection and Training

Based on our review, we identified potential challenges related to BHT selection and training. These are summarized in the following section.

Selection

Selection processes risk selecting BHTs that may lack fit with the job. Each service uses a somewhat different selection process, with varying strengths. For example, the Air Force requires completion of an MMPI-2-RF prior to entering the training pipeline, likely to ensure that candidates are suitable from a mental health perspective, as well as an entry interview. The Army requires BHTs attain an ASVAB Skilled Technical score of at least 101—the scale combines language, science, mathematics, and mechanical knowledge (U.S. Army, 2017b). Although these measures are an important first step in determining suitability for the career field, this test does not assess skills or characteristics that are more specific to the BHT career—for example, ability or comfort working in a profession that requires substantial face-to-face contact with other individuals, or interpersonal sensitivity and ability to demonstrate empathy. Another potentially important factor to consider is student interest in behavioral health. Ideally, students entering the career pipeline have some interest in behavioral health. However, there are other demands that may make it challenging to fulfill this requirement. For example, the number of authorized BHT positions in each service increased from fiscal years 2009 to 2012, suggesting growth in this field (U.S. Department of Defense, 2012); however, recent data from the Navy indicated that the proportion of BHTs to available billets was 76.2 percent, suggesting a shortage in available BHTs (Navy Personnel Command, 2018). Therefore, it may be more challenging to incorporate student interest as a formal selection criterion.

Training

The volume of material covered in the curriculum makes it challenging to address topics essential to clinical practice in much detail. The METC curriculum is designed to be comprehensive: incorporating all topics that students may need to be familiar with to perform the role of a BHT, providing opportunities for hands-on practice during coursework, and allowing for a brief applied clinical practicum experience. Therefore, instructors face the challenge of covering a breadth of material while trying to ensure enough depth of experience that students are prepared to enter a clinical setting.

Though the curriculum aims to provide students with a broad background, it is unclear how closely the curriculum reflects the experiences they will have once they enter the behavioral health workforce. Our review of the student guides for the consolidated courses suggested that each course provides high-level information about a range of relevant topics, but that this can limit the amount of detail on any given topic. For example, while the Psychopathology course broadly covers DSM-5 diagnoses, they are covered in an 85-hour time frame, and some diagnoses are seen infrequently in practice settings. For example, though approximately 7 percent of active-duty service members were diagnosed with adjustment disorders in 2016, 4 percent with depression, and 2.5 percent with PTSD, (Deployment Health Clinical Center,

2017), other disorders have less acute symptoms (e.g., certain neurocognitive disorders) and therefore may be encountered less in practice settings. This also limits time spent on diagnoses seen more frequently in clinical practice and curtails going into more depth on these diagnoses (e.g., providing multiple case examples, allowing opportunities to practice making a differential diagnosis, discussing how response to treatment may be assessed over time using measurement-based care), though this would likely have more relevance to clinical practice. BHTs are most likely to achieve the goal of increasing efficiency and efficacy of behavioral health services if they are well-versed in the diagnoses they will encounter most often.

Similarly, the Introduction to Counseling course provides a brief introduction to many types of theoretical orientations, though only a few are commonly used in clinical settings. This limits time that can be spent on practices used commonly in clinical settings (e.g., cognitive behavioral therapy [CBT]) (Hepner et al., 2017) and teaching students to implement specific evidence-based interventions consistent with their role at MTFs (e.g., problem solving therapy, motivational enhancement therapy).

Integration of interactive and applied exercises to teach course material can vary across instructors. Most of the material covered in the curriculum lends itself to being taught through various applied exercises. This could include case studies and vignettes, videos, and two-instructor role-play demonstrations. However, based on our discussions with students and instructors, there is a fair amount of instructor discretion in the use of these activities. Moreover, our review of the student guides demonstrated that there are few case examples incorporated in written materials. Best practices in training mental health professionals suggest the importance of opportunities to apply the course material, such as providing case examples that mirror what BHTs may encounter in clinical settings or modeling clinical skills (e.g., Beidas and Kendall, 2010).

Having practical components to certain courses, including the interviewing, counseling, and psychological testing courses, provides students with opportunities to practice skills learned in coursework. Live observation with real-time or near–real-time feedback can be an effective method of teaching clinical skills and is often used as part of clinical education programs, and the practical assessments do provide the opportunity for instructors to perform live observations of students performing clinical activities. However, given the pace of courses, students may have little opportunity to observe an "ideal" intake or counseling session—for instance, as demonstrated by two instructors—prior to attempting the skill themselves. There are also few templates or tools provided to students to structure these interactions. Though the clinical practicum at the end of the course provides another opportunity for hands-on practice of course material, limited supervisor availability places constraints on the amount of clinical contact students can have with patients, as does the brief length of the practicum.

Summary

This chapter reviewed the qualifications necessary to enter the BHT career field in each service branch. We also described the content and nature of the BHT curriculum, including the consolidated and service-specific courses and the directed clinical practicum, as well as the qualifications and training of instructors. We also discussed some of the key challenges related to selection and training of BHTs. In the next chapter, we describe the placement of BHTs following the completion of training at the METC, followed by a review of the roles and responsibilities that BHTs fulfill in garrison and in deployed or operational environments.

CHAPTER THREE

Behavioral Health Technician Roles and Responsibilities

After completing their training at the METC, BHTs become part of the behavioral health workforce. They may be assigned to a variety of settings, including clinical settings at MTFs (e.g., outpatient or inpatient clinics) or as part of an embedded behavioral health team. Once they enter the workforce, BHTs are expected to be prepared to perform a wide range of clinical tasks, including screening and assessments, intervention, case management, and outreach and prevention. In deployed or operational settings, their responsibilities have the potential to expand further. Their responsibilities may also expand or evolve as they progress through the levels specified in their branch of service. In this chapter, we describe the roles and responsibilities that BHTs may fulfill, both in garrison and in deployed or operational settings. We also review expectations for supervision and ongoing professional development. These descriptions are based on our review of relevant policy, as well as the literature review, supplemented by key informant discussions.

Placement of Behavioral Health Technicians Following Training

The assignment decisions for BHTs are made early during training, within the first several weeks. For example, Army students we spoke to during our visit to the METC had found out about their placement around their third week. Available placements are based on current staffing needs within a given service branch—that is, what medical centers, clinics, and/ or units have open billets. One key informant discussion suggested that the Army fills U.S. Army Forces Command (FORSCOM) positions first (i.e., operational billets), followed by U.S. Army Medical Command (MEDCOM) positions. The specific clinical setting is a decision made at the installation level, such that staff at the installation determine where to place a BHT. In medical settings, larger clinics may have more variety in the available placements (e.g., both inpatient and outpatient billets). In the Air Force, one key informant suggested that the decisions are based on staffing, though rank and level also play a role, as well as the specific capabilities needed at a given location. Therefore, if an open position requires someone with a particular skill set (e.g., Certified Alcohol and Drug Counselor [CADC] certification), it would not be filled by a BHT who has just completed the METC training. Most of the mental health workforce is in outpatient settings, so most BHTs begin in outpatient placements. In the Navy, one key informant suggested that placement decisions are similarly made based on staffing needs. The METC staff submit the names of Navy students for billet availability; these are sent to a career counselor and then to a detailer, who determines where BHTs are needed. Placement decisions are typically made based on their METC performance, with students per-

Figure 3.1
Placement Options Following Completion of the METC Training

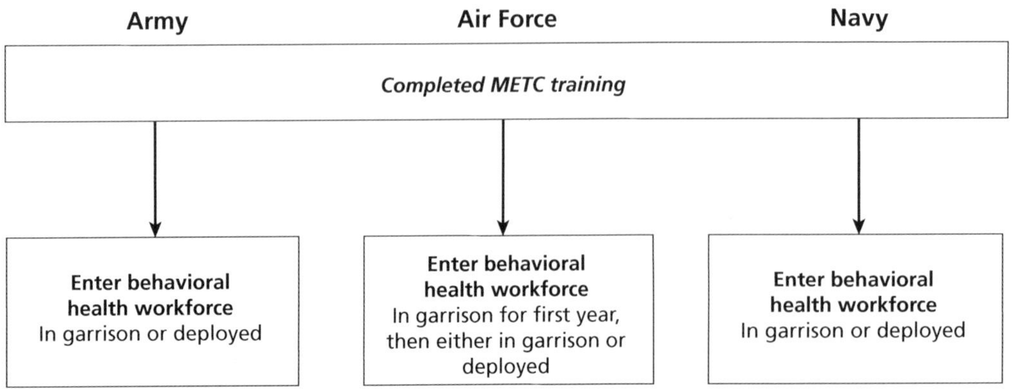

forming at the top of their cohort given first selection of available billets. An overview of BHT placement options by service branch appears in Figure 3.1.

BHT career progression varies from service to service. For example, in the Army, there are four skill levels for BHTs (Headquarters, Department of the Army, 2017b). Each skill level has a specific set of tasks that a service member is expected to be able to complete, with more managerial and administrative duties expected as skill level increases. There are also decreasing requirements for annual face-to-face contact hours as service members progress through skill levels (e.g., 750 required hours for skill level 1 vs. 200 hours for skill level 4) (U.S. Department of the Air Force, 2015; Headquarters, Department of the Army, 2017a; U.S. Air Force, 2017). In the Air Force, BHTs begin at the 1-level ("Helper") and are upgraded to the 3-level ("Apprentice") when they complete training at the METC. This qualifies them to perform certain tasks without supervision, provided that the tasks have first been conducted under "eyes-on" supervision by a mental health provider and received sign-off. For upgrade to the 5-level ("Journeyman"), BHTs must have a certain level of clinical experience and complete required Career Development Courses (CDCs), described in more detail later. For upgrade to the 7-level ("Craftsman"), BHTs must complete required CDCs and obtain their CADC certification. The highest level is the 9-level ("Superintendent"), which requires management experience. We did not identify information specific to the career levels of Navy BHTs.

BHT Roles and Responsibilities in Garrison

Most BHTs are placed in clinical settings at MTFs, though some BHTs are placed in embedded behavioral health positions in operational units, with the goal of expanding access to behavioral health care and reducing barriers to care (Carabajal, 2011; Losey, 2017; Russell et al., 2014; U.S. Army, 2013b). Though there can be variability in the specific activities BHTs complete depending on their assignment, BHTs are expected to potentially fulfill a wide range of roles and responsibilities. This includes not only clinical responsibilities, but also administrative and unit responsibilities. In the next section, we describe these in more detail.

Clinical Responsibilities

BHTs are expected to fulfill a range of clinical roles, depending on the nature of their placement. BHTs may be placed in inpatient or outpatient behavioral health clinics, drug and alcohol clinics, or as part of a Behavioral Health Optimizing Program (BHOP) collaborative care team alongside primary care providers (Air Force Instruction 44-121, 2018; Hoyt, 2017; Institute of Medicine, 2010; Nielson, 2016). We reviewed a number of policy documents describing the expected roles of BHTs across service branches, including the Army *Soldier's Manual and Trainer's Guide* (Headquarters, Department of the Army, 2017b) and *AFSC 4C0X1 Mental Health Service Specialty Career Field Education and Training Plan* (U.S. Department of the Air Force, 2015). We also reviewed job analyses (Air Education and Training Command Occupational Analysis Division, 2017), forms for rating clinical competencies (Headquarters, Department of the Army, 2017a), and job duty task analyses (U.S. Navy, 2013) to better understand expected roles across services. Based on this review, we identified four broad categories of clinical responsibilities, described in more detail next. Note that although these categories describe the potential range of clinical responsibilities that BHTs fulfill, the actual set of clinical responsibilities assigned to a BHT will depend on the clinic setting, as well as factors such as supervisor preference and other clinic demands (Carlton, 1979; Harris and Berry, 2013).

Screening and Assessment

BHTs play several roles related to screening and assessment. One such role includes conducting initial intake assessments and triaging patients (Headquarters, Department of the Army, 2017b; Hoyt, 2017; U.S. Air Force, 2017). As described, intake assessments are a key part of the training curriculum. Intake assessments include components such as identifying the patient's presenting concerns, assessing mental status, and conducting a risk assessment (i.e., determining risk of harm for self or others) (Headquarters, Department of the Army, 2017b; U.S. Air Force, 2017). In addition to gathering necessary data, BHTs are also responsible for being able to identify and communicate the patient's risk level and clinical needs to the licensed provider staffing the case. Though this generally would occur in a clinic setting in which the BHT would have the opportunity to meet in person with the licensed provider to discuss the case, there are also situations in which this intake and triage process may take place via telebehavioral health. For example, Garcia and Lindstrom (2014) described a context in which BHTs used telebehavioral health to expand the geographic reach of embedded behavioral health services. An embedded BHT accompanied their designated unit to a training site away from the main installation, while the embedded licensed providers were at the main installation. When mental health issues emerged, the BHT conducted an intake or triaged the patient in person and then discussed the case with the licensed providers via telebehavioral health to develop a treatment plan.

BHTs may also participate in the administration of psychological screening instruments and tests. This includes symptom screening measures (e.g., PTSD Checklist [Weathers et al., 2013]), personality assessments (e.g., MMPI-2 [Butcher et al., 2001]), cognitive and neuropsychological assessments (e.g., Hopkins Verbal Learning Tests–Revised [Brandt and Benedict, 2001]), intellectual assessments (e.g., Wechsler Adult Intelligence Scales–IV [Wechsler, 2008]), and achievement tests (e.g., Wide Range Achievement Test–Revised [Jastak and Wilkinson, 1984]) (Air Education and Training Command Occupational Analysis Division, 2017; Headquarters, Department of the Army, 2017b; U.S. Navy, 2013). BHTs may also be responsible for scoring these assessments, whether by hand or via computer (Air Education and Training

Command Occupational Analysis Division, 2017), though testing data and scores are then passed to a licensed provider for interpretation and feedback.

Psychosocial Interventions

BHT involvement in psychosocial interventions encompasses a range of activities. During their training, BHTs learn to implement brief, solution-focused interventions as part of their Counseling course (Headquarters, Department of the Army, 2017b; U.S. Air Force, 2017). Our discussions with key informants suggested that these are largely targeted toward individuals who present with psychosocial concerns (e.g., relationship difficulties), rather than patients with formal mental health diagnoses. BHTs also implement psychoeducational groups (Air Education and Training Command Occupational Analysis Division, 2017), and some documents suggest that they perform group counseling as well (U.S. Department of the Air Force, 2015; U.S. Navy, 2013).

BHTs may also provide alcohol and drug counseling (Air Education and Training Command Occupational Analysis Division, 2017). This is a particular focus in the Air Force, given its requirement that all BHTs become CADCs as part of their upgrade to the 7-level. Once certified, CADCs may perform some functions independently where allowed and as directed by the ADAPT Program Manager (PM) (Air Force Instruction 44-121, 2018), including counseling (*What Are the 12 Core Functions of a Drug and Alcohol Counselor?*, 2018), though some activities (e.g., initial assessment, treatment planning) are still performed under the supervision of a licensed provider (Air Force Instruction 44-121, 2018).

Case Management

BHTs may also be expected to participate in case management activities. At its most basic level, case management can include coordinating referrals for patients (U.S. Department of the Air Force, 2015; Headquarters, Department of the Army, 2017b). BHTs may also be involved in development of and assessment of progress through treatment plans, especially for those patients to whom they are providing counseling, including developing treatment goals, identifying treatment modalities, and evaluating the effectiveness of the treatment plan and modifying it as needed (Air Education and Training Command Occupational Analysis Division, 2017; Headquarters, Department of the Army, 2017b; U.S. Air Force, 2017). In addition, BHTs may play a role in medication management, including informing patients about prescribed medications, assessing medication adherence, and monitoring medication effects (including adverse and therapeutic effects) (Air Education and Training Command Occupational Analysis Division, 2017; Headquarters, Department of the Army, 2017b; U.S. Navy, 2013).

Outreach, Prevention, and Resilience

In addition to the clinical activities just described, BHTs have certain roles providing outreach and preventive services. In the military treatment facility (MTF) context, BHTs may be involved in consultation to non–behavioral health clinical settings. The BHOP program provides one example of this. BHOP integrates mental health providers into primary care teams; one potential role of BHTs in this setting is to conduct an initial assessment of patients before they see the licensed provider to determine the next steps and appropriate intervention (Nielson, 2016).

In addition, BHTs may have primary responsibilities related to outreach and resilience when they are embedded in an operational unit. For example, they may consult with unit leaders and members on topics relevant to behavioral health (U.S. Air Force, 2017) and help to assess behavioral health needs within a unit (Headquarters, Department of the Army, 2017b; U.S. Navy, 2013). BHTs may also be involved in providing pre- and postdeployment briefings and screenings for individuals new to an installation (Crossen, 2015). At some installations, they participate in the process of screening new trainees, or in pre- and postdeployment screenings. In these situations, individuals who express behavioral health concerns may be seen next by a BHT for an in-person interview to further assess behavioral health needs (Appenzeller, Warner, and Grieger, 2007; Garb et al., 2013; Srinivasan and DiBenigno, 2016). BHTs may also provide resilience programs, such as the Army Battlemind training (Appenzeller, Warner, and Grieger, 2007).

Administrative Responsibilities

Although BHTs are intended to serve as care extenders and fulfill clinical roles, a common concern expressed by key informants was that BHTs are often relied on for administrative responsibilities. These administrative responsibilities can include answering phones, scheduling patients, and records management. They can also include more clinically-relevant administrative tasks, such as coordinating hand-offs for patients with mental health needs (e.g., at a permanent change of station). In addition, BHTs may be tapped to perform facility-level tasks, such as overseeing a prevention program, performing accreditation-related tasks, and serving as training monitors or inspection control monitors. Depending on factors such as the clinic setting, availability of other administrative staff, and the specific supervisor to which a BHT is assigned, the amount of time spent in administrative versus clinical activities can vary substantially. For example, a study of BHTs working in BHOP found that the proportion of time spent on clinical responsibilities ranged from 10 percent to 75 percent (Nielson, 2016). In turn, the time spent in clinical versus other activities can have important implications—this study found that BHTs involved in more direct patient care reported higher job satisfaction and higher deployment readiness. This is also consistent with the findings of the Defense Task Force on Mental Health, which found that "technicians are being underutilized, often spending their time performing clerical tasks rather than the therapeutic support roles for which they were trained and which they are expected to exercise competently while deployed" (U.S. Department of Defense Task Force on Mental Health, 2007, p. 47). The Task Force formally recommended that BHTs be used to the full extent of their skills and training.

There have been some efforts to ensure that BHTs do not overly focus on administrative and clerical activities. For example, the Army mandates a certain number of client contact hours for each skill level—750 hours for skill level 10, 600 hours for skill level 20, 350 hours for skill level 30, and 200 hours for skill level 40 (Headquarters, Department of the Army, 2017a). That said, only 50 percent of this time must be spent in face-to-face activities; time spent in documentation or test scoring also qualifies as client contact hours. It is also important to note that, as BHTs get promoted, their time spent in managerial activities also increases. This accounts for the decreasing requirements for client contact hours outlined in Army policy (Headquarters, Department of the Army, 2017a). Based on our key informant discussions, though senior BHTs may maintain a small case load, they also are involved in activities such as training less experienced BHTs or assisting with clinic management.

Unit Responsibilities

In addition to their clinical and administrative responsibilities, BHTs must fulfill certain unit and military responsibilities. These can include motor pool, overnight staff duty, and charge of quarters assignments (Hoyt, 2017). Hoyt (2017) proposed a memorandum of understanding with a BHT's unit commander as a way to formally establish expectations for military versus clinic duties. This type of agreement could outline the time BHTs are expected to spend in clinic, as well as the specific unit missions that the BHT will participate in (e.g., company physical training, marksmanship ranges). However, it is not clear that these types of formal agreements are established with regularity to ensure that BHTs have sufficient time to spend in the clinical setting.

Roles and Responsibilities While Deployed or in Operational Settings

BHTs can deploy as part of medical units and may also deploy as part of operational units (Chappelle and Lumley, 2006; Hoyt, 2017; Peterson, Baker, and McCarthy, 2008). In the next section, we describe the roles of BHTs in deployed and operational settings, including their roles in medical and operational units.

Medical Units

BHTs can deploy as part of medical units, such as expeditionary medical units and combat stress control units (Chappelle and Lumley, 2006; Hall, 2009). In these contexts, BHTs work closely alongside licensed mental health providers, including psychiatrists, psychologists, social workers, and advanced practice psychiatric nurses.

In the Army, BHTs may serve as part of COSC detachments. In this role, they may staff restoration centers as part of a larger group of behavioral health providers and BHTs (Dailey and Ijames, 2014; Jones et al., 2013; Judkins and Bradley, 2017). Restoration programs are generally 24- to 72-hour programs for service members experiencing a combat operational stress reaction, providing life skills classes (e.g., resiliency, anger management, problem solving), occupational therapy, and time for leisure or physical activity (Smith-Forbes, Najera, and Hawkins, 2014) with the ultimate goal of returning the service member to duty. Some restoration programs also offer outpatient programs (e.g., Smith-Forbes, Najera, and Hawkins, 2014). In these programs, BHTs may conduct intake and follow-up assessments or facilitate life skills classes (Potter et al., 2009; Smith-Forbes, Najera, and Hawkins, 2014) and potentially provide individual therapy, depending on the severity of a case (Potter et al., 2009). BHTs who are members of COSC detachments may also split into smaller teams, typically comprising one mental health provider and one to three BHTs, allowing them to visit units stationed in the field (e.g., at forward operating bases) (Dailey and Ijames, 2014; Jones, Hammond, and Platoni, 2013; Jones et al., 2013). In these situations, these small COSC teams may be integrated with a forward operating base unit, and the BHT may perform activities such as informal outreach, teaching psychoeducational groups (e.g., stress management), and conducting intakes as needed for licensed providers (DeCoster, 2014; Jones et al., 2013). These smaller teams might also be tapped to provide services to units after a traumatic event; a COSC team might be sent to a forward operating unit to deliver debriefings and provide support as needed (DeCoster, 2014; Jones, Hammond, and Platoni, 2013).

In the Air Force, BHTs may have roles providing care at Air Force theater hospitals and expeditionary medical hospitals. For example, Peterson, Baker, and McCarthy (2008) described mental health care provided at an Air Force theater hospital and contingency aeromedical staging facility in Iraq. At the Air Force theater hospital, one BHT worked alongside two licensed providers, supporting behavioral health care—including a role in consultation with medical patients, though the specific role of BHTs in this context was not described. At the contingency aeromedical staging facility, two BHTs worked with a mental health nurse, with the goal of screening patients and preparing for aeromedical evacuation. Chapelle and Lumley (2006) described care provided at an Air Force outpatient mental health clinic, part of an expeditionary medical hospital in Iraq, which was manned by a team of one psychologist or psychiatrist and one BHT for three-to-four-month periods. Care provided included psychological evaluation and triage, psychiatric hospitalization, and outpatient treatment and follow-up, with a focus on brief intervention. The literature also described the role of BHTs in providing preventive care as part of a medical company ("Embedded Airmen Aid Camp Taji Troops," 2009). In this instance, mental health providers were responsible for providing more formal treatment, while BHTs focused on preventive interventions.

Operational Units

BHTs may also deploy as part of deployed operational units. Like BHTs who are embedded in units in garrison, these BHTs are assigned to serve the needs of the operational unit of which they are a part.

In the Army, one example of BHTs deployed as part of an operational unit is the BHTs embedded in Stryker Brigade Combat Teams. When serving as part of an embedded behavioral health team, they may be responsible for outreach and consultation to a large population; for example, an article described how the Mental Health Section of one Stryker Brigade Combat Team was assigned one behavioral health provider and one BHT for more than 5,000 soldiers in 13 locations, and coverage had to be augmented by a medical unit (Doboszenski, 2005). In addition to performing typical duties of embedded behavioral health providers, including outreach and consultation, BHTs deployed as part of an operational unit may also help to extend the geographic reach of services. For example, Hoyt and colleagues (2015) described behavioral health services provided by a behavioral health team embedded in a Stryker Brigade Combat Team, including two licensed behavioral health providers and three BHTs. The licensed providers were placed at the larger medical facility in the region, while BHTs were assigned to forward battalion aid stations. In this case, BHTs helped to provide telebehavioral health, with the BHT sitting in the room with the service member during consultation while connected to the licensed provider via webcam. The provider would formulate a plan, and the technician would help to implement this plan and follow up with the patient while the patient continued to have regular sessions with the provider. This extended the reach of behavioral care across a greater geographic region.

Navy BHTs embedded in operational units have the potential to serve multiple types of roles. For example, they may be embedded with a Marine Expeditionary Unit as part of the Operational Stress Control and Readiness program (Knight, 2012). In this context, mental health providers and BHTs serve as combat stress control professionals rather than clinical health care providers. More specifically, BHTs may be involved in activities such as leading psychoeducational classes and providing information on topics such as warning signs of stress-related problems.

Navy BHTs may also be part of behavioral health teams embedded in units on Navy ships, such as aircraft carriers (Johnson, Ralph, and Johnson, 2005). In addition, recent pilot programs have been implemented to embed mental health providers into U.S. Submarine Forces (Miletich, 2017; Rapley et al., 2017). These programs are located at the nearby naval station or waterfront clinic, with the goal of providing "easier access" to psychological support (Rapley et al., 2017, p. e1676), and even send mental health providers to submarines to determine whether there are mental health concerns (Miletich, 2017). In one such program, located on the East Coast of the United States, the embedded behavioral health team comprised one full-time and one part-time mental health provider and one BHT (Rapley et al., 2017). This pilot program was found to increase the number of sailors served and the proportion of sailors returning to duty after seeking psychological care. A similar program located in the Pacific region has been associated with a decreased wait time for services (Miletich, 2017). Our key informant discussions suggested that Navy BHTs can also help to bridge geographic divides in this context; for example, an amphibious ready group may have a licensed mental health provider on the largest ship in the group and send BHTs to the smaller ships within the group to provide in-person coverage.

Supervision

Because BHTs are not credentialed providers (with the exception of Air Force 7-level BHTs, who are CADCs), they work under the supervision of licensed mental health providers. Our discussions with key informants highlighted that supervisors generally include psychiatrists, clinical psychologists, licensed clinical social workers, and advanced practice psychiatric nurses. Depending on the organization of a given clinic, a BHT may have a primary supervisor or receive oversight from multiple supervisors.

There is limited policy guidance related to supervision requirements for BHTs. A recent Army policy memo indicates that BHTs must be "under the direct supervision of a licensed and/or privileged provider, appropriate to the duties assigned"; however, specific requirements are not described (Headquarters, Department of the Army, 2017a). The Air Force outlines certain requirements for upgrade at each level. For example, 3-level BHTs must be trained and task certified before they can perform a task unsupervised; however, even when a BHT is working unsupervised, a licensed mental health provider must have direct contact with the patient "of sufficient length and interaction to validate the assessment and recommendation" (U.S. Department of the Air Force, 2015). There are also specific supervision requirements for BHTs who are CADCs, who must be observed and assessed at least twice per month, totaling at least two hours (Air Force Instruction 44-121, 2018). Though BHTs can perform a number of tasks independently once they become CADCs, initial assessment, treatment planning, and crisis intervention must be performed under supervision (Air Force Instruction 44-121, 2018).

Some MTFs have spearheaded efforts to formalize the provision of supervision. For example, during our key informant discussions, we learned of two large MTFs that have training programs for mental health providers (e.g., psychiatry and psychology residents). Providers and senior BHTs at these sites have built in supervision of BHTs as a specific learning experience for provider trainees. This not only offers mental health provider trainees valuable experience with supervision, but it also ensures that BHTs receive a standard amount of supervision and helps mental health providers better understand the capabilities and skills of BHTs. However, our analyses of available sources suggest that these types of efforts are not standard and not systematically available across training sites.

Ongoing Training and Professional Development

Although the METC provides a foundation of knowledge and skills, the expectation is that BHTs will participate in ongoing training and professional development activities. There are some service-specific policies designed to support ongoing skill development.

Our key informant discussions suggested that much of the ongoing professional development of BHTs takes place in the form of on-the-job training (OJT), though it is likely that the nature of this OJT may vary based on location and supervisor preference. In addition to OJT, the services promote more structured ongoing training opportunities, such as self-studies or online courses. Based on our key informant discussions and policy review, it appears that the Air Force has the most standardized continuing education requirements. As part of an airman's upgrade to 5-level and 7-level, Air Force BHTs must complete CDCs. These home-study courses consist of fundamental information that airmen are expected to know before moving to the next career stage (U.S. Department of the Air Force, 2015).

Air Force BHTs must also fulfill specific requirements to maintain CADC certification, including continuing education as required for recertification, which takes place every three years (Air Force Instruction 44-121, 2018). In our key informant discussions, this certification was often cited as a significant asset, as it not only ensured ongoing professional development but also provided Air Force BHTs with a tangible output of their efforts and helped providers have more confidence in their skill level.

Although other services have continuing education requirements (e.g., the Army requires 12 hours annually of "accumulative study in the [behavioral health] field, either in a class, a self-study course, or in-service training"), these are not based on a standard body of knowledge or competencies that are expected of BHTs. However, there may still be expectations for the maintenance of specific skills. For example, the Army has a competency checklist of specific skills that BHTs must be able to demonstrate to a supervisor on an annual basis, with increasing competencies expected at increasing skill levels (Headquarters, Department of the Army, 2017a).

Key informant discussions suggested that BHTs may have some ability to attend local and national conferences as part of their ongoing professional development. One key informant also suggested that there are some Army-wide centrally funded courses (e.g., traumatic event management, motivational interviewing); however, some may have a specific rank requirement, so not all BHTs are eligible to attend. During our key informant discussions, we also learned that some clinical sites have developed educational curricula for their behavioral health technicians. For example, a provider at a large MTF established a training syllabus for BHTs, which includes topics such as informed consent, assessing risk, and elements of a treatment plan. The syllabus also covers specific therapeutic techniques, such as progressive muscle relaxation, sleep hygiene, and use of thought records to address cognitive distortions. While licensed mental health providers at MTFs may have latitude to create these types of learning experiences, our synthesis of available information suggested that they are not standard across MTFs or across services.

Key Challenges

BHT Roles and Responsibilities in Garrison

BHTs require OJT to develop their skills, but there appears to be no standard expectation as to how OJT should be specifically operationalized, build on the METC training in a meaningful way, and be widely disseminated and implemented in an effective and standardized manner. BHTs are expected to fulfill a wide range of clinical roles once they enter the behavioral health workforce. Though BHT training focuses on a broad range of topics, the complete BHT training course is only 14 to 17 weeks in length, depending on the service, with limited opportunities to practice clinical skills in classroom or practicum settings. In part, this means that significant OJT is needed once BHTs enter the workforce, which, according to key informant discussions, requires an investment of time on the part of the licensed mental health provider(s) with whom the BHT works. That said, based on our discussions, it is unclear whether providers understand the time needed to help BHTs develop the clinical skills that would make them most effective in a given clinical setting, whether they know enough about the curriculum to understand how to build on the core set of skills that BHTs have been taught, or whether they are afforded the time necessary to engage in BHT training.

It is also important to note that there is no existing civilian model on which BHT roles, responsibilities, and OJT can be modeled. Though there are civilian psychiatric technicians, their roles tend to be more circumscribed than that of the BHT, and there is no formal licensing, credentialing, or certification process. Though the credentialing for licensed mental health providers generally requires specific levels of OJT (as well as supervision), their training is so much more intensive in duration and scope that it can be challenging to consider how those expectations could be adapted for BHTs.

BHTs are not consistently used to the full extent of their clinical training, and there is a need to better understand how factors such as the setting, supervisor preferences, and clinic administrative demands affect their roles to determine how they can be used more effectively. There are also concerns as to whether BHTs are being used to the full extent of their training. It is likely that several factors may contribute to this issue. For example, the settings in which BHTs are placed may affect the types of opportunities that are available to them. The preferences and style of the supervisor may play a role, including level of comfort delegating tasks to BHTs, understanding of BHTs' clinical skills, and the model used to integrate BHTs into the clinic workflow. For example, some providers may prefer to have BHTs conduct the initial triage for a patient but want to be present or take the lead on all future clinical contact (e.g., intake and treatment); other providers may be willing to have BHTs work more autonomously, providing brief interventions for individuals who present with less significant psychosocial concerns. BHTs working with a provider with the latter preference may in turn have better-developed intervention skills. The administrative demands of the clinic may also play a role; for example, clinics without dedicated administrative support may rely more on BHTs to complete administrative support tasks. Though it may be appropriate for BHTs to be responsible for some administrative tasks in this situation, a BHT who spends 75 percent of his or her time on administrative tasks has very limited opportunity to practice, hone, and maintain clinical skills. However, without formal guidance as to the amount of time that BHTs should spend engaged in clinical activities, it may be challenging for clinics to know what the alternatives are, or to spend time carving out protected time for BHTs. In turn, this is a concern because future assignments—particularly those in deployed or operational settings—may hinge on the expectation that BHTs are prepared to complete all tasks learned at the METC, not just a subset of these tasks.

Deployed and Operational Settings

It is unclear whether and to what extent BHTs are prepared to fulfill the roles expected of them, especially in deployed or operational settings. BHTs may serve in different types of units and different types of roles when in deployed or operational settings. Regardless of the position, though, a key theme across our key informant discussions and literature review was that the responsibilities of BHTs can expand substantially under these circumstances. Our review of the literature suggests that many of the specific clinical tasks that BHTs complete while deployed or operational are similar to the tasks they may complete in garrison (e.g., intake assessments, outreach, psychoeducational groups); however, they may be responsible for providing services to a much larger population of service members and appear to work very closely with a single mental health provider. They also have opportunities to work more autonomously; for example, when serving to extend the geographic reach of mental health services, a BHT may be the only behavioral health representative in a given location or on a given ship. Even if such a BHT connects regularly with a licensed mental health provider to staff cases, this is still a greater degree of autonomy than a BHT may experience while at an MTF.

It remains unclear whether BHTs are prepared for this expanded level of responsibility or autonomy when they deploy. Though our follow-on survey will provide more detailed information about this question, concerns about deployment readiness were raised during our key informant discussions. More specifically, when BHTs are used largely for administrative or clerical tasks in garrison, they may have limited opportunities to practice and hone the skills they need while deployed (U.S. Department of Defense Task Force on Mental Health, 2007). Moreover, though the Air Force requires at least one year of garrison experience prior to deployment, BHTs from the Army and Navy may be deployed or placed in operational settings as their first position following the METC. Though these BHTs would have completed a clinical practicum before completion of the METC, the practicum provides minimal clinical experience. Because the METC is designed to provide a foundation of skills that are further developed by OJT, BHTs who deploy immediately after the METC must do that on-the-job learning in an environment with a high operational tempo, and in which the pace of clinical responsibilities may make it challenging for the licensed mental health provider to invest substantial time in the ongoing professional development of BHTs with whom they deploy.

Supervision, Ongoing Training, and Professional Development

There is limited guidance governing specific expectations or requirements for supervision, ongoing training, and professional development of BHTs. Because BHTs are unlicensed, they are supposed to complete their work under the supervision of a licensed mental health provider. This may include providing services together (e.g., jointly conducting an intake, with both parties asking questions), having the licensed mental health provider observe the clinical encounter without actively participating unless a specific concern arises, having the BHT discuss the case with a licensed mental health provider after the interaction, or having the licensed mental health provider meet briefly with the patient following patient interaction with a BHT. However, the extent to which these various modes of supervision serve as a learning experience for the BHT can vary greatly. For example, if a licensed mental health provider meets with the patient to ensure that the BHT's assessment of clinical needs and risk is valid, it ensures the quality of services provided to the patient but may not directly help a BHT know how to improve upon their clinical skills. There is little formal guidance regarding expectations for supervision of BHTs (e.g., recommended frequency or intensity of supervision), nor formal training or guidance to supervisors on how to most effectively supervise BHTs, which may lead to differences in skill development across supervisors or assignments. To some extent, variability in the degree of supervision may be appropriate, depending on the specific responsibilities of a BHT in a given setting; however, especially if minimum expectations for clinical practice are established, developing a minimum expectation for supervision would be beneficial as well.

Similarly, there are few structured requirements related to ongoing training and professional development. The Army has set expectations related to annual continuing education activities, and the Air Force has developed specific CDCs that must be completed upon upgrade to each level. These are important starting points for establishing standard expectations for ongoing training. As mentioned before, the METC curriculum is relatively brief, with the expectation that skills will be honed once BHTs enter the workforce—but because the specific responsibilities of a BHT can vary so substantially based on the clinical setting, clinic demands, and supervisor preferences, the lack of standardized ongoing training opportunities means that BHTs may have uneven opportunities to grow in their knowledge and skills.

In turn, the lack of standardization in supervision and ongoing training is a concern because licensed mental health providers may expect BHTs to have a certain set of skills based on their METC training; however, without ongoing training and professional development, BHTs may have weaknesses in certain areas. Our key informant discussions suggested that licensed mental health providers may be less likely to assign clinical responsibilities to BHTs if they have concerns about their level of training or skills; these may be situations that lead to BHTs being tasked with administrative responsibilities. In addition, uneven knowledge and skill development at one assignment may mean that a BHT is unprepared for the responsibilities expected at the next assignment, which can be a particular concern in deployed settings.

Summary

This chapter provided a review of the roles of BHTs once they enter the behavioral health workforce, beginning with their first duty assignment following completion of the METC. In addition to describing the range of clinical and other activities that BHTs are expected to perform, we discussed how roles may change in the deployed or operational environment. We also reviewed requirements related to supervision, ongoing training, and professional development. Finally, we discussed challenges faced by BHTs in clinical settings, including their level of preparedness to fulfill the roles expected of them and the lack of structured requirements for professional development. In the next chapter, we discuss potential solutions for addressing the challenges identified in Chapter Two and Chapter Three.

CHAPTER FOUR

Summary and Recommendations

BHTs have an important role in the military behavioral health workforce. Specifically, they are intended to be care extenders, with the goal of expanding access and improving the quality of services provided to service members. In the previous chapters, we provided an overview of the selection, training, and professional roles of BHTs. BHTs receive a broad educational foundation, spanning the knowledge and skills deemed to be relevant to their work in a number of settings. This comprehensive curriculum combines didactic and practical components, including the opportunity to practice skills in a clinical practicum setting. After completion of training, they go on to play roles in a number of settings, ranging from MTFs to embedded behavioral health teams, and from garrison to deployed or operational environments. While conducting this review, we identified certain key challenges to the effective training and use of BHTs. In this chapter, we describe potential recommendations to address the key challenges that were identified.

Summary of Key Challenges

In Table 4.1, we summarize the key challenges described in the previous chapters.

Recommendations to Guide Improvements in the Selection, Training, and Use of Behavioral Health Technicians

Recommendation 1. Establish a Consistent Set of Selection Criteria to Ensure Fit with the Career Field

Currently, each service branch uses somewhat different selection criteria. While service branch differences may be appropriate to some extent, as they reflect the priorities and expectations for BHTs in a given branch of service, it would likely be beneficial to establish some minimum standard. For example, the Air Force requires an entry interview before beginning BHT training. Though it was unclear what the focus of that interview is currently, it may be possible to build upon this practice and develop a structured entry interview template that all services could use as a gateway to the training pipeline. This interview could cover topics that are already considered by the services, such as suitability for the career from a medical and behavioral health perspective. It could also be expanded to assess interest in behavioral health. It would likely also be beneficial to incorporate some type of assessment of interpersonal skills; though it is possible to teach some of the skills that are important to the provision of behav-

Table 4.1
Summary of Key Challenges to the Effective Training and Use of BHTs

Domain	Key Challenge
Selection	• Selection processes risk selecting BHTs that may lack fit with the job.
Training	• The volume of material covered in the curriculum makes it challenging to cover topics essential to clinical practice in much detail. • Integration of interactive and applied exercises to teach course material can be variable across instructors.
BHT roles and responsibilities in garrison	• BHTs require OJT to develop their skills, but there appears to be no standard expectation as to how OJT should be specifically operationalized, build in a meaningful way on the METC training, and be widely disseminated and implemented in an effective and standardized manner. • BHTs are not consistently used to the full extent of their clinical training, and there is a need to better understand how factors such as the setting, supervisor preferences, and clinic administrative demands affect their roles to determine how they can be used more effectively.
Deployed and operational settings	• It is unclear whether and to what extent BHTs are prepared to fulfill the roles expected of them, especially in deployed or operational settings.
Supervision, ongoing training, and professional development	• There is limited guidance governing specific expectations or requirements for supervision, ongoing training, and professional development of BHTs.

ioral health, such as demonstrating empathy, it is helpful if a candidate has some baseline level of interpersonal sensitivity, comfort, and interest in working with others. Personnel selection research indicates that interviews are especially effective when they are structured and suggests the utility of strategies such as situational interviewing (i.e., asking a candidate to explain how they would handle a situation relevant to the BHT career [Robertson and Smith, 2001]). Establishing a minimum standard for selection across services would also be beneficial for settings in which BHTs from multiple services work alongside one another, such as large MTFs.

It is important to note that the ways in which certain selection criteria are used was unclear (e.g., the MMPI-2-RF results in the Air Force), and we did not find any efforts to validate whether these criteria are effectively screening for disqualifying factors. It would be beneficial to have a better understanding of how these criteria are used and the extent to which current selection criteria are identifying candidates who are a good fit for the career, which would then inform more specific recommendations. For example, to determine whether ASVAB scores are an effective way of identifying appropriate and successful candidates, it would be useful to conduct a formal validation study to ascertain the extent to which ASVAB scores are predictive of outcomes such as academic performance at the METC or job performance once in clinical settings (Cassenti, Rice, and Rose, 2015; Held et al., 2015).

In addition, data about the ways that service branches differ in their use of BHTs would help to guide any further recommendations about whether selection criteria should be identical across services or, perhaps, have certain common elements while allowing for service-specific variability. Moreover, the reorganization of medical services under the Defense Health Agency may provide an opportunity to harmonize aspects of the BHT career, including selection criteria, so it will be important to consider the extent to which this would be beneficial.

Recommendation 2. Align the Curriculum with Demands of BHTs in the Field and with the Needs of the Population They Serve

Recommendation 2a. Focus the Curriculum on the Conditions BHTs Encounter Most Often

The instructors at the METC are faced with the challenge of covering a significant amount of material in a relatively short period of time. Currently, the curriculum is set by reviewing the core competencies expected of BHTs in each service and then ensuring that the curriculum covers topics relevant to these competencies. That said, there may be opportunities to better align the curriculum with the roles BHTs play in the field and tailor the curriculum to the population they serve.

Although there is value in reviewing all DSM-5 diagnoses in detail, the Psychopathology course is one of the lengthiest BHT courses. Moreover, BHTs may encounter certain categories of diagnoses very infrequently in clinical settings. One option may be to focus the Psychopathology course on the diagnoses seen most often in clinical settings (e.g., the most common ten to 15 diagnoses). This strategy would have several advantages. First, focusing on a smaller set of diagnoses would allow instructors to devote more time to case vignettes and other applied examples. For example, time could be spent reviewing multiple case examples to demonstrate nuances of how certain disorders may manifest in different patients. Exercises could also be incorporated to help BHTs learn how to make a differential diagnosis in instances in which a patient presents with symptoms that may be shared by multiple diagnoses, assess clinical improvement over time, and assess response to treatment and/or side effects. Not only can these types of active learning strategies improve understanding of the material, but these types of case examples and activities would prepare BHTs to know what types of follow-up questions they may need to ask when conducting an intake assessment in a clinical setting to better understand a patient's presenting concern, establish patient-centered goals, and assess progress at any subsequent encounters.

Recommendation 2b. Create Standardized Training Tools That Will Translate to Practice

Though students receive guides for each of their courses, there may be additional opportunities to incorporate standardized tools for training. For example, during the Interviewing Skills course, students learn the specific categories of information that they are expected to cover as part of an intake assessment. As part of the didactic component of this course, students could be provided with a standard intake assessment form. This would have several potential advantages. First, this template could be used to incorporate demonstrations into the coursework. For example, two instructors could each demonstrate how they might use the intake assessment form during an initial meeting with a patient. This would allow students to see how the intake assessment form could be used to gather information in a systematic way and the ways that clinicians may frame the same question differently depending on personal style or the responses of the client. Second, this intake assessment form could be used in the practical/laboratory components of the course and, ultimately, when students graduate and enter the workforce. Though they could tailor the instrument to their own needs once they enter the clinical setting, it would create a foundational standard for intake assessments across BHTs, ensuring that all BHTs have learned to collect the most critical pieces of information from patients during an intake session. This recommendation is also consistent with the recommendation of Hoyt (2017), who suggested that templates, checklists, and similar resources are a way to standardize BHT practice. That said, it is also important to consider that some individual supervisors or clinics may have their own templates or specific areas they want covered during an intake; therefore, BHTs may also benefit from training in adapting their baseline template to meet the expectations of different supervisor or clinic demands, to prepare BHTs for success in a range of assignments.

Recommendation 2c. Teach a Core Set of Evidence-Based Interventions That Generalize to Many Clinical Settings or Patient Populations

Currently, the Introduction to Counseling course provides an overview of many psychotherapy techniques—but the curriculum largely provides a theoretical overview rather than education about how to implement any particular modalities. Students then learn to conduct a counseling session, which includes components of goal-setting and problem-solving but is not necessarily anchored in theory. However, when they enter clinical settings, they are likely to encounter CBT more often than the other therapeutic techniques discussed in the class and, in some cases, may be expected to implement CBT-based interventions. To bridge this gap between the classroom and practice, one option may be to focus the counseling component of the curriculum on a subset of specific, solution-oriented interventions that can be implemented for many presenting concerns and patient populations, such as problem-solving therapy or motivational enhancement therapy. These approaches share many elements of the current counseling principles that students learn (e.g., identifying goals, brainstorming ways to meet goals, reviewing pros and cons for potential solutions) but have the advantage of being anchored in theory. These approaches also lend themselves to the use of worksheets, which can be a valuable tool for structuring clinical interactions. Moreover, incorporating specific evidence-based practices of this nature into the curriculum would allow instructors to use validated measures of fidelity to ensure that students reach adherence and competence in the delivery of an intervention (Institute of Medicine, 2015).

Similarly, students learn how to practice leading psychoeducational groups, but the coursework is not structured around specific topics that may be commonly covered. Instead, students could learn to implement a core set of common psychoeducational groups (e.g., sleep hygiene, stress management, smoking cessation), which could cover a standard set of topics and include evidence-based worksheets and activities.

In turn, the clinical practicum at the end of the METC training would provide students with the opportunity to begin to apply these interventions in a clinical setting. There are still limitations to the amount of practice students may get, due to the brevity of the practicum experience and limited availability of supervisors, but having a core set of interventions to practice during this experience may be a way to maximize the time students spend on practicum.

We acknowledge that teaching these types of interventions may be more time-consuming or require more course preparation than some of the existing approaches taught in the curriculum. Therefore, it would be important to evaluate whether current staffing at the METC can support this type of recommendation.

That said, this approach would not only ensure that BHTs are prepared for the settings in which they will be placed but would also have advantages for their supervisors. In particular, supervisors would know that all newly trained BHTs are equipped with a core set of individual counseling skills and know how to facilitate a specific set of psychoeducational groups and, therefore, may better know how to maximize their involvement in clinical activities (versus more administrative activities). Supervisors could also continue to use fidelity assessments to ensure the ongoing quality of clinical services provided by BHTs.

Recommendation 3. Standardize Expectations for Involvement in Clinical Activities and Ongoing Training, Clinical Supervision, and Professional Development in the Field
Recommendation 3a. Establish Training Plans for BHTs Entering New Clinical Settings

As described previously, there are no standardized efforts across service branches to provide OJT and additional training for BHTs entering new clinical settings. The Air Force Career Field Education and Training Plan for BHTs describes task qualification requirements that are needed for advancement to the next skill level, which must be formally documented (U.S. Department of the Air Force, 2015); similarly, the Army has an annual competency assessment for BHTs (Headquarters, Department of the Army, 2017a). We also learned that some MTFs have made efforts to develop training curricula for BHTs to build upon their training at the METC. These curricula are an effort to ensure that BHTs have the background and experiences necessary to be successful in the given setting. These types of extended training programs are sometimes used in civilian contexts to improve the integration of care extenders into clinical settings. For example, Will and colleagues (2010) described a training program for new physician assistants in a hospital setting. This program involved the physician assistants completing a series of two- to four-week rotations in different areas of the hospital over a one-year period, which was supplemented with didactics, lectures, and self-directed modules, as well as formal competency assessments during each rotation. It would be challenging to implement a training program this intensive for BHTs in their first clinical setting; however, a potential adaptation may be to build in a six- to 12-week training experience at the beginning of any new placement to provide a more in-depth introduction to the clinical setting. This would be valuable for BHTs in their first clinical placement and for BHTs who are placed in a new setting (e.g., moving from outpatient to inpatient). Less intensive versions of this type of training experience could also be adapted. For example, Hull and colleagues (2013) described a training and career ladder for medical assistants, through which they developed three trainings for new medical assistants. These were completed at various intervals (e.g., within the first week, between six months and one year) and incorporated small-group instruction, demonstration, and then assessments of medical assistant skills. This type of course was found to have a positive effect on clinical skills.

A structured training experience of this nature would require additional investment on the part of licensed mental health providers—and potentially senior BHTs—when new BHTs arrive in a given setting. However, this upfront investment in training could ultimately save providers time if they feel more comfortable sharing clinical duties with BHTs. This type of training could also augment the METC curriculum by teaching clinical activities specific to the setting or the needs of the patient population. For example, this type of training has been used in civilian contexts to expand the potential roles of medical care extenders, allowing them to participate more in preventive activities and health coaching or assist with outreach to high-need patients (Naughton et al., 2013). This would also build on existing efforts by the services to incorporate educational experiences, such as the Air Force CDCs, in a way that is more hands-on and tailored to the needs of the specific setting.

The Navy uses a personnel qualification standards (PQS) program to implement this type of structured training experience for hospital corpsmen completing "A" school (U.S. Department of the Navy, 2017). At their first duty assignment at an MTF, new corpsmen must demonstrate proficiency on a standard set of skills. The completion of the PQS must be documented, but, in addition, commanding officers are required to "develop a rotational plan of various clinical areas to provide hospital corpsmen the broadest access to patient encounters to meet PQS completion requirements" (U.S. Department of the Navy, 2017), p. 3). This PQS program is not required of corpsmen who complete specialized training, including BHTs; however, this is a potential foundation upon which training plans for BHTs in new clinical settings could be built.

Establishing these types of training plans for BHTs entering new clinical settings would likely facilitate the integration of BHTs into clinical tasks, as licensed mental health providers would have more confidence regarding the baseline level of skill of their BHTs. That integration, in turn, would ensure that BHTs are maximally effective as care extenders.

Recommendation 3b. Develop Requirements for Specific Clinical and Educational Experiences

BHTs require substantial OJT and clinical experience to build on the foundation of skills gained at the METC; however, their involvement in clinical activities may be limited by other responsibilities, such as administrative tasks, and there are few requirements related to clinical experience or ongoing training. In turn, this has implications for the readiness of BHTs when they deploy or are placed in operational settings, during which time their involvement in clinical activities can expand greatly.

Because the clinical responsibilities of a BHT can be so specific to a setting or supervisor, there is the potential for great variability in the clinical experiences that BHTs have. In addition, being placed in a clinic with high administrative demands may result in the BHT having limited clinical involvement. However, this means that when BHTs deploy, it may have been some time since they have engaged in the specific clinical activities commonly expected of them in deployed or operational environments (e.g., intakes, psychoeducational groups, counseling sessions). To ensure the readiness of BHTs, it could be beneficial for each service to identify a core set of skills that it expects of BHTs while deployed or operational, and then build in requirements related to those skills to be fulfilled in garrison. For example, if intakes are seen as a critical task of BHTs, there may be a requirement that BHTs complete at least one intake per month in garrison, regardless of setting. This would ensure that BHTs maintain some baseline level of skill on those critical tasks. At the moment, it is unclear to what extent BHTs have the opportunity to maintain proficiency in the clinical skills required most commonly in deployed and operational settings, nor what those skills may be; however, our survey will provide additional context for expanding on this recommendation.

Similarly, the services could consider centering their requirements for continuing education around these topics. For example, the Air Force requires the completion of CDCs for upgrade to each skill level. If a specific clinical skill or knowledge area were considered critical for deployment (e.g., combat operational stress reactions), it could be flagged as a recurring topic to appear in the CDCs. Though the Navy and Army do not appear to have the same type of standard continuing educational experience, they could institute similar requirements (e.g., that ongoing education must touch on certain topics). This is commonly done for credentialing of providers—for example, many states require clinical psychologists to complete a certain number of continuing education hours related to ethics (e.g., California Code of Regulations, 2013; Pennsylvania Psychological Association, 2018; West Virginia Board of Examiners of Psychologists, 2018). These types of requirements are also used in the ongoing credentialing of civilian medical care extenders—for example, the Certifying Board of the American Association of Medical Assistants requires that individuals either recertify via examination (to demonstrate core knowledge) or complete continuing education to include general, administrative, and clinical content areas that align with medical assistant competencies (American Association of Medical Assistants, 2018; Certifying Board of the American Association of Medical Assistants, 2018).

Finally, only the Air Force requires BHTs have at least one year of experience in garrison prior to deployment. This ensures that BHTs have had the opportunity to employ their clinical skills outside the METC setting. This is likely a requirement that would be beneficial across services to ensure the readiness of deployed and operational BHTs.

Recommendation 3c. Establish Requirements or Guidance for Effective Supervision

Our review of policies related to supervision revealed the lack of guidance regarding the necessary or recommended frequency or intensity of supervision. Because BHTs are expected to continue to develop the clinical skills learned during their training at the METC through OJT, supervision is an important consideration. Our key informant discussions suggested that providers may supervise in many ways, including through direct observation of clinical work, cofacilitating intake sessions or psychoeducational groups, and staffing of cases after BHTs engage with patients one-on-one. Though these experiences all provide opportunities for BHTs to be given feedback and learn through observation, the lack of policy guidance means there can be substantial variability in time spent on supervision. As with the previous recommendation, our follow-on survey will provide additional context for expanding on this recommendation.

Another key consideration is the content of supervision. In a recent position paper on the education, training, and supervision of neuropsychological test technicians (also known as psychometrists), the National Academy of Neuropsychology highlighted that supervision should touch on a range of topics, including the specific assessment procedures being implemented (e.g., tests, scoring systems) and ethics and confidentiality (Puente et al., 2006). Similarly, guidance for the supervision of peer support specialists in the civilian sector has highlighted the importance of discussing not only job performance but also career development (Cabral et al., 2014). When supervision is provided only as part of direct observation of clinical encounters or when staffing clinical encounters, there may be limited opportunities to provide supervision focused on these broader topics. Establishing a regular schedule for meeting with BHTs to provide supervision may create opportunities to discuss not only performance of clinical skills but also bigger-picture concepts relevant to BHTs (e.g., how clinical skills in garrison translate to deployed settings; recent research relevant to the roles of BHTs).

Recommendation 4. Consider Drawing from Best and Innovative Practices in the Civilian Sector for Incorporating Care Extenders into Clinical Care

One challenge that providers and clinics may face is understanding the most effective way to incorporate BHTs so that they truly act as care extenders, increasing efficiency, access, and quality of care (Schendel, 2018). A given clinical setting may have a mix of different licensed mental health providers, with little formal guidance outlining the best workflow to provide efficient and effective care. Therefore, understanding how to integrate BHTs in a way that promotes efficiency and effectiveness may be challenging. The ideal model for integrating BHTs may depend on the specific setting and its workflow and the needs of its patients. To determine the best way to integrate BHTs into the workflow of a clinic, a starting point might be to understand the range and/or epidemiology of the kinds of conditions being seen and how providers are employed in treating these conditions. These factors would then guide the types of roles that BHTs should fulfill to increase the efficiency and effectiveness of behavioral health care in the military. Ultimately, this would allow the military to design a system that meets the needs of the military population and operates at the highest levels of quality with maximum efficiency.

That said, there are practices that can be drawn from civilian care extender models. A model that is commonly used to integrate medical assistants into primary care settings is the "teamlet" model. This generally involves a licensed clinician working with one or two medical assistants (Bodenheimer and Laing, 2007; Bodenheimer and Willard-Grace, 2016). In this model, the medical assistant helps to streamline the provision of care through three main steps. First, before seeing a patient, there is generally a meeting between the clinicians and medical assistant to review the clinical goals for the patient. The medical assistant is then the first to see the patient in a *previsit*, during which the assistant may take a medical history, review medications, and preview the goal of the visit. The clinician then joins, leading the visit, while the medical assistant documents the encounter. Finally, the medical assistant closes out the visit with the patient in a *postvisit* phase, in which the assistant reviews the visit with the patient, makes sure that the patient knows next steps, and assists in goal setting. The medical assistant may also be involved in between-visit care, such as checking in with patients with more chronic conditions. This model bears some resemblance to the ways that we heard BHTs are sometimes used in clinical settings, with the BHT conducting the initial intake; staffing the case with the licensed provider; and then determining who will follow up on the treatment plan, given the nature and severity of the presenting concern.

Increasingly, civilian care extenders are being used as part of patient education and chronic disease management, in a health coach–type role. For example, medical assistants may be taught strategies related to behavior change facilitation, such as motivational interviewing, allowing them to check-in with patients and help to assess and promote progress toward the treatment goals (Chapman and Blash, 2017; Ladden et al., 2013; Nelson et al., 2010). In these models, medical assistants remain in close contact with the patients' providers—for example, via a daily huddle, in which the medical assistant provides an update to the licensed clinician, and the clinician can identify patients who may be in need of more intensive services (Nelson et al., 2010). This is another model that could be adapted for the BHT context; for example, if BHTs were trained in problem-solving therapy or motivational enhancement therapy, as described previously, they would be well-suited to address the ongoing needs of patients who may have less severe presenting concerns (e.g., those presenting with psychosocial concerns rather than formal diagnoses). The facilitation of psychoeducational groups would also be consistent with this type of patient education model.

Finally, the civilian literature describes increasing instances in which care extenders are provided with supplemental training to increase their effectiveness in a specific clinical setting. This involves serving in roles ranging from care coordinator or patient navigator to quality improvement assistant (Blash, Chapman, and Dower, 2011; Chapman and Blash, 2017). As described in Recommendation 3a, the establishment of a training plan for BHTs entering a new clinical setting may provide the opportunity to train BHTs on any additional responsibilities that would be appropriate for their backgrounds and helpful to the clinic. These types of additional professional development activities can also be beneficial for care extender satisfaction (Naughton et al., 2013).

Limitations

Although this report provides important background for understanding the use of BHTs as part of the military behavioral health workforce, there are also important limitations to our findings. First, our review was based on the policy and curriculum documents that were available to us. Though we made an effort to identify as many relevant documents as possible, both via searches of relevant websites and through discussions with key informants, there are certain documents we may not have been aware of or may not have been able to access. That said, this may also suggest the need to make certain expectations for BHT training and roles and responsibilities more explicit (e.g., by incorporating them into guidance and policy documents).

Second, although we conducted key informant discussions, they included a small number of informants and were focused on providing additional context for the policy and curriculum documents. It would be informative to conduct in-depth interviews with a broader range of BHTs and licensed providers to gain a more detailed understanding of the variability in how BHTs are used across services and settings. We were also limited to visiting the METC training campus, though site visits of behavioral health and other clinical settings across services would also yield valuable information.

Finally, though we were able to describe the range of activities that BHTs may engage in, we understand that there is substantial variability in the field. Ideally, the BHT curriculum will closely align with the roles expected of BHTs in the field. Though our review of policy documents gave us an initial understanding of the range of roles that may be expected, these were quite broad, and it is difficult to know the extent to which these roles and responsibilities are actually expected and carried out in the workforce. We were also unable to capture any differences related to training needs and roles/responsibilities for active-duty service members compared with those in the National Guard or Reserve forces. Similarly, our review of documents also provides limited basis for identifying potential barriers to optimizing the role of BHTs, and therefore for identifying potential solutions. These are topics that will be covered on our follow-on survey of BHTs and licensed mental health providers, which will provide important data about the ways that BHTs are actually being used in practice, their preparedness for fulfilling these roles, and the barriers that may prevent them from being used most effectively. In that way, it is likely that our understanding of key challenges will expand significantly after fielding the survey, and that there will be opportunities to make more specific and data-driven recommendations. For example, the data may help us to better evaluate whether common job descriptions across service branches would be appropriate, or whether there are enough service-specific differences to warrant unique job descriptions and responsibilities. If the data suggest that standardization of core competencies across service branches is warranted, then recommendations related to the establishment of a certification or credentialing program may also be considered.

Summary

This report provides an overview of the selection, training, and roles and responsibilities of BHTs. Our goal was not only to document the BHT career trajectory, but also to understand obstacles to optimizing the use of BHTs as care extenders in the military. In addition to providing a description of each of these phases of a BHT's career, we have identified key challenges at each stage. We also reviewed potential recommendations that could address these challenges, drawing from our understanding of the military behavioral health context and from best and innovative practices in the use of civilian care extenders. Therefore, this report provides our initial insights on ways to more effectively use BHTs and a foundation for the surveys of BHTs and licensed mental health providers that are the next step in this project.

Policy and Curriculum Documents Reviewed

As part of this study, we conducted a review of relevant policies across service branches. We also identified documents related to the education and training of BHTs, both at the standardized curriculum level and at the installation level. This appendix catalogs the types of documents we reviewed and brief descriptions of each document.

Policy Documents

To understand what policies exist regarding BHTs in the military, we reviewed policy documents from each service branch. These documents are categorized by service branch in Tables A.1–A.3.

Curriculum Documents

To better understand the initial training completed across services, we received documents relevant to the curriculum completed by all BHTs at the METC in San Antonio, Texas (Table A.4).

During our key informant discussions, we also learned of local efforts to structure ongoing training for BHTs once they enter the workforce. Key informants shared the documents listed in Table A.5, which are components of these installation-level approaches to train or assess BHTs.

Table A.1
Army Policy Documents

Document Title	Publication Date or Effective Date	Description
Soldier's manual and trainer's guide MOS [Military Occupational Specialty] 68X, Behavioral Health Specialist	April 28, 2017	A training and skills guide for Army BHTs
MOS 68X Utilization Matrix	No date	A matrix of Army BHT tasks and skill levels created at Womack Army Medical Center
Force Health Protection Field Manual (ATP 4-02.8)	March 9, 2016	Force Health Protection doctrine for support to unified land operations
Combat and Operational Stress Control Field Manual (FM 4-02.51)	July 6, 2006	Outlines the functions and operations of each COSC element within an area of operations; provides guidance for COSC support
OTSG/MEDCOM Policy Memo 15-041 Military Occupational Specialty 68X, Behavioral Health Specialist Utilization	July 27, 2015 (Expired: July 17, 2017)	Policy memo issued in July 2015 describing how BHTs must be utilized and what competencies must be maintained while serving in a BH capacity; expired July 2017
OTSG/MEDCOM Policy Memo 17-080 Military Occupational Specialty 68X, Behavioral Health Specialist Utilization	December 28, 2017 (Expiration: December 28, 2019)	Policy memo issued in December 2017 describing how BHTs must be utilized and what competencies must be maintained while serving in a BH capacity; expires December 2019
CMF 68 Smartbook	October 1, 2018	Prerequisites, qualifying scores, and other requirements for 68 MOS
68X Competency Assessment	April 14, 2015	Rubric for annual assessment of BHT competencies

Table A.2
Air Force Policy Documents

Document Title	Publication Date or Effective Date	Description
Air Force Instruction 44-121 Alcohol and Drug Abuse Prevention and Treatment (ADAPT) Program	July 18, 2018	Guidance for the USAF Alcohol and Drug Abuse Prevention and Treatment Program, including USAF policy regarding alcohol abuse, prescription drug misuse, and drug abuse
AFSC 4C0X1 Mental Health Service Specialty Career Field Education and Training Plan	February 15, 2015	Training plan for USAF mental health specialists, including skill levels, training requirements, and career field information
Career Detail: "Mental Health Service"	May 1, 2017	Detailed description of the duties, responsibilities, and training of the 4CO1X (mental health specialist) position
4C0X1 Job Analysis	June 2017	Analysis of duty areas and tasks performed by USAF behavioral health technicians
Air Force Instruction 44-172 Mental Health	November 13, 2015	Instruction on implementing Air Force mental health policies

Table A.3
Navy Policy Documents

Document Title	Publication Date or Effective Date	Description
BUMED Instruction 1510.23D Hospital Corpsman Skills Basic	May 17, 2015	Instruction establishing guidelines, training requirements, and competencies for hospital corpsmen
Instructor requirements for Navy Medicine Training Support Center		Standards and requirements for instructors at the Navy Medicine Training Support Center
HM NEC Manning Snapshot May 2018	May 2018	Provides detail about the proportion of billets that are filled for all hospital corpsman specialties
MILPERSMAN 1910-120 Separation by reason or convenience of the government—physical or mental conditions.	March 15, 2012 Cancelled	Policy and procedures on separating Navy service members from the service due to physical or behavioral conditions that impair their performance
Chapter 12, Education and Training, in *Manual of the Medical Department.*	November 1, 2016	Chapter on education and training of Navy medical officers and enlisted personnel
CANTRAC Volume II	Published annually	Includes details of Navy training courses, including the purpose and scope of courses, prerequisites, and eligibility requirements
Job Duty Task Analysis Management Manual	2013	Description of specific duties and tasks conducted by Navy mental health technicians; released in 2013
Instruction on Hospital Corpsman Personnel Qualification Standards Program	October 11, 2017	BUMED instruction on the competencies and qualifications of hospital corpsman personnel
Personnel Qualification Requirements for Hospital Corpsman	August 2017	Description of the PQS program for hospital corpsman personnel; describes the system of validating minimum level of competency in certain areas prior to performing duties, as well as explaining the required competencies and duties
Hospital Corpsman Career Roadmap	January 2018	Roadmap that describes a hospital corpsman's trajectory through the Enlisted Learning and Development Continuum, the curriculum and process to become a sailor and corpsman

Table A.4
METC Curriculum Documents

Document Title	Publication Date or Effective Date	Description
Air Education and Training Command, *Course Training Plan L5ABJ4C031 01AA (PDS Code LBI) Mental Health Service Apprentice*. Course training plan L5ABJ4C031 01AA (PDS Code LBI) Mental Health Service Apprentice	2015	Overview of training and courses for behavioral health technicians at the METC
2017–2019 General Catalog Number 21	May 11, 2017	Air University at Community College of the Air Force's course catalog; includes CCAF policies and degree programs and requirements
Medical Education and Training Campus (METC) Behavioral Health Technician Program Curriculum Plan	November 18, 2015	Detailed description of the behavioral health technician training program, including courses, course descriptions and objectives, branch-specific courses, and clinical practicum
Behavioral Health Specialist, Behavioral Health Technician, Mental Health Service Apprentice Resource Requirements Analysis Report	June 24, 2015	Report on resources required for BHT programs across service branches; includes curriculum information, information about current BHT classes, instructor requirements, and facility requirements
Consolidated Course Schedule	2017	Sample course schedules for classes of BHTs at the METC

Table A.5
Installation-Level Approaches to Ongoing Training of BHTs

Document Title	Publication Date or Effective Date	Description
Lackland Air Force Base		
ADAPT Welcome Letter	April 4, 2018	Welcome letter for BHTs selected to rotate through the ADAPT program at Lackland
ADAPT 90-day Training Rotation Schedule	No date	Schedule of trainings and objectives for ADAPT trainees at Lackland Air Force Base CADC
CADC Written Case Presentation Plan	No date	Agreement for CADC trainee written case presentation plan and the supervision involved
Womack Army Medical Center		
68X Assessment Evaluation Questions	No date	Questions and scales used to assess 68X competencies at WAMC
68X Training Modules	No date	Breakdown of training modules for 68Xs; includes module titles, training topics, and assignments and activities
68X Training Program Briefing	No date	Briefing on the duties, utilization, training requirements, and training programs for 68Xs at Fort Bragg and WAMC
Initial Competency Assessment, Womack Army Medical Center: Behavioral Health Technician	April 14, 2015	Evaluation form for 68X competency assessments

Literature Review Search Terms

Uniformed Behavioral Health Technician Review

Preliminary searches indicated that peer-reviewed literature about military BHTs is limited; therefore, we searched both peer-reviewed and gray literature sources. This allowed us to identify documents that appeared in traditional academic journals, as well as documents that were not peer-reviewed but still provided relevant information about BHTs. To conduct a search of literature related to uniformed BHTs, we searched PsycINFO, Google Scholar, ProQuest Military Database, Defense Technical Information Center, the Congressional Research Service, and the National Academies Press.

Given the limited literature available on this topic, we conducted this search using terms used by each service branch to refer to the BHT profession (i.e., "behavioral health technician" and "mental health technician") and terms previously used by the services to refer to BHTs (e.g., "mental health service specialist"). We also used terms that describe the role of BHTs that may be used in civilian literature (e.g., "paraprofessional," "psychiatric technician," "care extender"); when these terms were used in the non–military-specific databases (i.e., PsycINFO, PubMed, Google Scholar, Congressional Research Service, National Academies Press), they were combined with the term "military" to ensure results were relevant to uniformed BHTs.

Given the limited literature available, we opted not to limit the search with more-specific terms, such as "training," "education," or "role," though our goal was to identify documents that provided information about these facets of BHT practice.

Specific search terms included the following:

- behavioral health technician
- allied health professional
- mental health technician
- behavioral health specialist
- mental health services apprentice
- behavioral science specialist
- mental health specialist
- mental health service specialist
- paraprofessional
- psychiatric technician
- psychiatry technician

- psych* technician
- psychiatr* tech*
- psychol* tech*
- psych tech
- care extender.

After we removed duplicates, the search returned 59 results. All 59 documents underwent a full text review, with sources determined to be relevant if they mentioned BHTs in any capacity. Of these sources, ten were screened out due to irrelevance, such as not discussing BHTs or not describing aspects of the MHS. The remaining 49 sources were included. Information was abstracted from these sources using a structured data abstraction form, which included information such as type of source, methodology, service branch(es) of focus, topic covered (e.g., role of BHTs in garrison, role of BHTs while deployed), and key findings. In addition, we supplemented the search with one blog post identified during the policy review and an article identified during a search of literature related to care extenders in civilian behavioral health settings (described later), for a total of 51 included documents.

In total, we reviewed 27 peer-reviewed journal articles, 13 non–peer-reviewed articles (for example, press releases or military magazine articles), eight reports, one historical report on Navy medical education and training, one U.S. Army Medical Department Center and School course catalog, and one thesis. Of these sources, 11 were specific to the Air Force, 27 to the Army, six to the Navy, and seven addressed more than one service branch.

Our review of these sources revealed that very few publications specifically focus on BHTs and their role in the military. The majority of sources (n = 38) described the role of BHTs as part of a larger team of behavioral health professionals in garrison, while deployed, and in other circumstances, such as disaster response. Though a subset of these sources detailed the roles that BHTs played within the behavioral health team, others did not elaborate on the BHT's specific role. Other topics covered by these sources included education and training of BHTs (n = 2), the history of BHTs in the military (n = 3), and the growth of the BHT workforce (n = 1). We also found a resource guide providing a crosswalk between military occupations and analogous civilian positions based on the Occupational Information Network (n = 1) (National Center for O*NET Development, undated). Four sources specifically addressed the role and utilization of BHTs within the military health care system; however, three of these were interviews or first-person anecdotal accounts, and only one was a peer-reviewed article.

Civilian Health Care Extender Review

Behavioral Health Settings

We also conducted a search of the literature related to individuals in the civilian sector who have roles as behavioral health care extenders. Our goal was to focus on individuals in professions who perform a similar scope of work. For careers specific to mental health, we conducted a search for the career term alone; for those not necessarily specific to mental health, we included a term to indicate that context.

To examine the civilian research related to care extenders in behavioral health setting, we searched PsycINFO and PubMed. Search terms included:

- psychiatric technician
- psychometrist
- peer specialist
- peer support specialist
- technician [any field] AND (behavioral health or mental health or psych* [title, abstract, subject, or keyword]) (PsycINFO)
- care coordinator AND (psychology OR mental health OR behavioral health [title, abstract, subject, keyword]) (PsycINFO)
- care manager AND (psychology OR mental health OR behavioral health [title, abstract, subject, keyword]) (PsycINFO)
- care coordinator[Title/Abstract] AND (psychology[MeSH Terms]) OR mental health [MeSH Terms] (PubMed)
- care manager[Title/Abstract] AND (psychology[MeSH Terms]) OR mental health [MeSH Terms] (PubMed).

After we removed duplicates, this search yielded 560 sources. Following a title/abstract review, 44 sources were retained. Articles were excluded during the title/abstract review if they did not relate to behavioral health care or did not appear to focus on the role of the care extender. A number of these articles were published before 1990 (n = 12); to ensure relevance to the current care systems and positions, we excluded these from our full text review. We conducted a full text review of the remaining 32 sources.

The goal of this search was to understand in what ways behavioral health professionals in the civilian workforce parallel the role and experience of BHTs in the military, and how these civilian roles might inform training and best practices for BHTs. Therefore, sources in the full-text review were included if they described the role or duties, training, or best practices for this kind of care extender. Using these criteria, 17 sources were identified as relevant with full texts available.

Of these sources, about one-third of them (n = 6) discussed the duties and roles of a care extender in a behavioral health environment. Other topics that these sources addressed included the capabilities of care extenders to implement interventions (n = 3), standards and credentialing (n = 2), training of behavioral health care extenders (n = 3), supervision (n = 1), and guidance for implementing the care extender role in a behavioral health setting (n = 2).

Other Medical Settings

To supplement the search of care extenders in civilian behavioral health settings, we also conducted a literature review of medical care extenders. After comparing the education, training, and responsibilities of various types of medical care extenders, we concluded that the positions of medical assistant and physician assistant most closely parallel the BHT position in the MHS. We selected medical assistants, given that the level of training received and role as a care extender is comparable to that of BHTs; we selected physician assistants because, although they can practice independently, the wide scope of skills and responsibilities expected of physician assistants parallels that of BHTs. The goal of this search was to understand how medical care extenders are trained on the job and supervised, as well as frameworks for integrating care extenders into medical clinics and recommended best practices for this integration.

Given the medical focus of this search, we conducted this search in PubMed, limiting the search to articles published after 1990. Our search strategy combined a term reflecting the clinicians of interest (medical assistants and physician assistants) with a term to reflect our focus on training, teaching, and roles of these care extenders.

Clinician search terms included

- medical assistants [Title/Abstract]
- physician assistants [MeSH Terms].

Terms to reflect training, teaching, and/or roles included

- ((teaching[MeSH Terms]) OR Education, Professional[MeSH Terms]) OR Staff Development[MeSH Terms]
  - For the search of the physician assistants literature, which was much larger, we further scoped this search by adding the term "AND model [Title/Abstract] OR framework [Title/Abstract]"
- professional role[MeSH Terms]
  - For the search of the physician assistants literature, which was much larger, we further scoped this search by adding the term "AND model [Title/Abstract] OR framework [Title/Abstract]"
- credential*[Title/Abstract]
- supervision[Title/Abstract].

After we screened for duplicates, 345 sources were returned. We conducted a title/abstract review to exclude sources that did not describe training, best practices, credentialing, or an implementation framework for care extenders. Forty-nine sources were identified for full-text review. Fifteen sources were screened out during full-text review because they did not cover the target topics, and four were unavailable despite efforts to reach out to the author. This search was supplemented by a targeted internet search of the gray literature, including the Learning from Effective Ambulatory Practices Program Primary Care Team Guide and Healthforce Center at University of California San Francisco, which yielded six sources. In total, 36 sources were reviewed. These included sources describing ways to integrate a care extender into a clinic or treatment team (n = 8), the skills and capabilities of a care extender and how those might be utilized innovatively (n = 13), supervision (n = 2), care extender credentialing and ways to assess competency (n = 5), OJT programs for care extenders (n = 7), and how to determine what patients can be treated by a care extender rather than a provider (n = 1).

References

Air Education and Training Command, *Course Training Plan L5ABJ4C031 01AA (PDS Code LBI) Mental Health Service Apprentice*, Randolph, Tex.: U.S. Air Force, 2015.

Air Education and Training Command Occupational Analysis Division, *Occupational Analysis Report Mental Health Services AFSC 4C0X1 OSSN 3056*, Joint Base San Antonio Randolph, Tex.: Air Force Occupational Analysis Program, 2017.

Air Force Instruction 44-121, *Alcohol and Drug Abuse Prevention and Treatment (ADAPT) Program*, 2018.

Air University, *2017–2019 General Catalog Number 21*, Maxwell Air Force Base, Ala., 2017. As of May 24, 2018:
https://www.airuniversity.af.edu/Portals/10/CCAF/documents/CCAF_2017_2019_General_Catalog.pdf

American Association of Medical Assistants, *CMA (AAMA) Recertification by Continuing Education Application*, application form, Chicago, Ill., 2018.

Appenzeller, George N., Christopher H. Warner, and Thomas Grieger, "Postdeployment Health Reassessment: A Sustainable Method for Brigade Combat Teams," *Military Medicine*, Vol. 172, No. 10, 2007, pp. 1017–1023.

Beidas, Rinad S., and Philip C. Kendall, "Training Therapists in Evidence-Based Practice: A Critical Review of Studies from a Systems-Contextual Perspective," *Clinical Psychology–Science and Practice*, Vol. 17, No. 1, 2010, pp. 1–30.

Blair, Bradley, and Pete Kelley, "Introduction of the Behavioral Health Technician Work Group," blog post, 2017. As of May 24, 2018:
http://www.pdhealth.mil/news/blog/introduction-behavioral-health-technician-work-group

Blash, Lisel, Susan A. Chapman, and Catherine Dower, *Workforce Collaborative Trains Medical Assistants to Enhance Care at Community Health Centers*, San Francisco, Calif.: UCSF Center for the Health Professions, 2011.

Bodenheimer, Thomas, and Brian Y. Laing, "The Teamlet Model of Primary Care," *Annals of Family Medicine*, Vol. 5, No. 5, September–October 2007, pp. 457–461.

Bodenheimer, Thomas, and Rachel Willard-Grace, "Teamlets in Primary Care: Enhancing the Patient and Clinician Experience," *Journal of the American Board of Family Medicine*, Vol. 29, No. 1, 2016, pp. 135–138.

Brandt, Jason, and Ralph H. B. Benedict, *Hopkins Verbal Learning Test–Revised. Professional Manual*, Lutz, Fla.: Psychological Assessment Resources, 2001.

Butcher, James N., John R. Graham, Yossef S. Ben-Porath, Auke Tellegen, W. Grant Dahlstrom, and Beverly Kaemmer, *MMPI-2: Manual for Administration and Scoring (Revised Edition)*, Minneapolis, Minn.: University of Minnesota Press, 2001.

Cabral, Linda, Heather Strother, Kathy Muhr, Laura Sefton, and Judith Savageau, "Clarifying the Role of the Mental Health Peer Specialist in Massachusetts, USA: Insights from Peer Specialists, Supervisors and Clients," *Health & Social Care in the Community*, Vol. 22, No. 1, 2014, pp. 104–112.

California Code of Regulations, Title 16, Division 13.1, Article 10, Continuing Education Requirements, § 1397.61, 2013.

Carabajal, Shannon, "Army Expanding Successful Embedded Behavioral Health Program," press release, 2011. As of May 24, 2018:
https://www.army.mil/article/69479/army_expanding_successful_embedded_behavioral_health_program

Carlton, Thomas G., "Navy Psychiatric Technicians in the Outpatient Setting," *U.S. Navy Medicine*, 1979, Vol. 70, pp. 17–19.

Cassenti, Daniel, Valerie Rice, and Paul N. Rose, "The Relationship Between U.S. Military Aptitude Testing and Academic Performance During Army Combat Medic Training," *Proceedings of the Human Factors and Ergonomics Society Annual Meeting*, Vol. 59, 2015, pp. 859–863. As of January 2, 2019:
https://journals.sagepub.com/doi/pdf/10.1177/1541931215591257

Certifying Board of the American Association of Medical Assistants, "CMA (AAMA) Recertification by Continuing Education Application," 2018. As of October 31, 2018:
http://www.aama-ntl.org/docs/default-source/recertification-by-continuing-education/recert-by-ce-app.pdf?sfvrsn=16

Chapman, Susan A., and Lisel K. Blash, "New Roles for Medical Assistants in Innovative Primary Care Practices," *Health Services Research*, Vol. 52, No. S1, 2017, pp. 383–406.

Chappelle, Wayne, and Vicki Lumley, "Outpatient Mental Health Care at a Remote US Air Base in Southern Iraq," *Professional Psychology: Research and Practice*, Vol. 37, No. 5, 2006, p. 523.

Clay, Derrick R., *Medical Education and Training Campus (METC) Behavioral Health Technician Program Curriculum Plan*, Joint Base San Antonio Fort Sam Houston, Tex.: Medical Education and Training Campus, 2016.

Crossen, Erica, *Reducing Stigma Through Outreach: A Mental Health Technician's Experience*, AF.mil, 2015.

Dailey, Jason I., and Victoria L. Ijames, "Evolution of the Combat and Operational Stress Control Detachment," *US Army Medical Department Journal*, 2014, pp. 8–13.

DeCoster, Vaughn, "Combat Social Work During the Surge in Iraq," *Social Work in Mental Health*, Vol. 12, No. 5–6, 2014, pp. 457–481.

Deployment Health Clinical Center, *Mental Health Disorder Prevalence Among Active Duty Service Members in the Military Health System, Fiscal Years 2005–2016*, Falls Church, Va.: Defense Centers of Excellence for Psychological Health and Traumatic Brain Injury Center, 2017. As of July 3, 2018:
http://www.pdhealth.mil/sites/default/files/images/mental-health-disorder-prevalence-among-active-duty-service-members-508.pdf

Doboszenski, Scot A., "Combat Health Support in the Army's First Stryker Brigade," *Army Logistician*, Vol. 37, 2005, pp. 4–9.

"Embedded Airmen Aid Camp Taji Troops," press release, U.S. Air Force, Camp Taji, Iraq, 2009.

Garb, Howard N., James M. Wood, Kristin Schneider, Monty Baker, and Wendy Travis, "Suitability Screening During Basic Military Training," *Military Psychology*, Vol. 25, No. 1, 2013, pp. 82–91.

Garcia, Michelle M., and Kristin J. Lindstrom, "Telebehavioral Health: Practical Application in Deployed and Garrison Settings," *U.S. Army Medical Department Journal*, October–December 2014, pp. 29–35.

Hall, J. Camille, "Utilizing Social Support to Conserve the Fighting Strength: Important Considerations for Military Social Workers," *Smith College Studies in Social Work*, Vol. 79, No. 3–4, 2009, pp. 335–343.

Harris, Jesse J., and Stacey Berry, "A Brief History of the Military Training of the Enlisted Mental Health Worker," *Journal of Human Behavior in the Social Environment*, Vol. 23, No. 6, 2013, pp. 800–811.

Headquarters, Department of the Army, *OTSG/MEDCOM Policy Memo 17-080, Military Occupational Specialty 68X, Behavioral Health Specialist Utilization*, Joint Base San Antonio, Fort Sam Houston, Tex.: Headquarters, U.S. Army Medical Command, 2017a.

———, *Soldier's Manual and Trainer's Guide MOS 68X, Behavioral Health Specialist*, Washington, D.C., 2017b.

———, "TRADOC Regulation 350-6: Enlisted Initial Entry Training Policies and Administration," 2017c. As of February 22, 2019:
http://adminpubs.tradoc.army.mil/regulations/TR350-6withChange1.pdf

Health Care Interservice Training Office, *Behavioral Health Specialist, Behavioral Health Technician, Mental Health Service Apprentice Resource Requirements Analysis Report*, Fort Sam Houston, Tex.: Medical Education and Training Campus, 2015.

Held, Janet D., Thomas R. Carretta, Sarah A. Hezlett, Jeff W. Johnson, Jorge L. Mendoza, Norman M. Abrahams, Fritz Drasgow, Rodney A. McCloy, and John H. Wolfe, *Technical Guidance for Conducting ASVAB Validation/Standards Studies in the U.S. Navy*, Millington, Tenn.: Navy Personnel Research, Studies, and Technology, 2015. As of October 31, 2018:
https://www.dtic.mil/dtic/tr/fulltext/u2/a612759.pdf

Hepner, Kimberly A., Coreen Farris, Carrie M. Farmer, Praise O. Iyiewuare, Terri Tanielian, Asa Wilks, Michael Robbins, Susan M. Paddock, and Harold Alan Pincus, *Delivering Clinical Practice Guideline–Concordant Care for PTSD and Major Depression in Military Treatment Facilities*, Santa Monica, Calif.: RAND Corporation, RR-1692-OSD, 2017. As of August 9, 2018:
https://www.rand.org/pubs/research_reports/RR1692.html

Hoyt, Tim, "Clinical Supervision and Management of US Army Behavioral Health Technicians," *Military Behavioral Health*, 2017, pp. 1–7.

Hoyt, Tim, Gustavo Garnica, Devin Marsh, Keri Clark, Jason Desadier, and Sterling Brodniak, "Behavioral Health Trends Throughout a 9-Month Brigade Combat Team Deployment to Afghanistan," *Psychological Services*, Vol. 12, No. 1, 2015, p. 59.

Hull, Tammie, Patricia Taylor, Emily Turo, Joan Kramer, Susan Crocetti, and Maura McGuire, "Implementation of a Training and Structured Skills Assessment Program for Medical Assistants in a Primary Care Setting," *Journal for Healthcare Quality*, Vol. 35, No. 4, July–August 2013, pp. 50–60.

Institute of Medicine, *Provision of Mental Health Counseling Services Under TRICARE*, Washington, D.C.: National Academies Press, 2010.

———, *Psychosocial Interventions for Mental and Substance Use Disorders: A Framework for Establishing Evidence-Based Standards*, Washington, D.C.: National Academies Press, 2015.

Jastak, Sarah, and Gary S. Wilkinson, *The Wide Range Achievement Test: Manual of Instructions*, Wilmington, Del.: Jastak Associates, 1984.

Johnson, W. Brad, John Ralph, and Shannon J. Johnson, "Managing Multiple Roles in Embedded Environments: The Case of Aircraft Carrier Psychology," *Professional Psychology: Research and Practice*, Vol. 36, No. 1, 2005, p. 73.

Jones, David E., Patricia Hammond, and Kathy Platoni, "Traumatic Event Management in Afghanistan: A Field Report on Combat Applications in Regional Command–South," *Military Medicine*, Vol. 178, No. 1, 2013, pp. 4–10.

Jones, David E., Franca Jones, Laura Suttinger, Ayessa Toler, Patricia Hammond, and Steven Medina, "Placement of Combat Stress Teams in Afghanistan: Reducing Barriers to Care," *Military Medicine*, Vol. 178, No. 2, 2013, pp. 121–125.

Judkins, Jason L., and Devvon L. Bradley, "A Review of the Effectiveness of a Combat and Operational Stress Control Restoration Center in Afghanistan," *Military Medicine*, Vol. 182, No. 7, 2017, pp. e1755–e1762.

Knight, Dustin, *15th MEU Receives Mental Health Provider*, press release, USS *Peleliu*, At Sea, 2012.

Ladden, Maryjoan D., Thomas Bodenheimer, Nancy W. Fishman, Margaret Flinter, Clarissa Hsu, Michael Parchman, and Edward H. Wagner, "The Emerging Primary Care Workforce: Preliminary Observations from the Primary Care Team: Learning from Effective Ambulatory Practices Project," *Academic Medicine*, Vol. 88, No. 12, 2013, pp. 1830–1834.

Losey, Stephen, "New in 2018: New Mental Health Programs Seek to Ease Strain on Airmen, Families," *Air Force Times*, 2017. As of May 24, 2018:
https://www.airforcetimes.com/news/your-air-force/2017/12/27/new-in-2018-new-mental-health-programs-seek-to-ease-strain-on-airmen-families/

Medical Education and Training Campus, *Behavioral Health Technicians*, Fort Sam Houston, Tex.: Defense Health Agency, 2018a. As of May 24, 2018:
http://www.metc.mil/academics/BH/

———, *Medical Education and Training Campus*, Fort Sam Houston, Tex.: Defense Health Agency, 2018b. As of May 24, 2018:
http://www.metc.mil/

METC—*See* Medical Education and Training Campus.

Miletich, Derek, *COMSUBPAC Embedded Mental Health Program (eMHP)*, blog post, Joint Base Pearl Harbor–Hickam, Hawaii: Submarine Force Pacific, U.S. Navy, 2017. As of May 24, 2018:
https://www.csp.navy.mil/Blog/Blog-Post/Article/1113830/
comsubpac-embedded-mental-health-program-emhp/

National Center for O*NET Development, O*NET OnLine, online tool, U.S. Department of Labor Employment and Training Administration, undated. As of February 22, 2019:
https://www.onetonline.org/

Naughton, Dana, Alan M. Adelman, Patricia Bricker, Michelle Miller-Day, and Robert Gabbay, "Envisioning New Roles for Medical Assistants: Strategies from Patient-Centered Medical Homes," *Family Practice Management*, Vol. 20, No. 2, 2013, pp. 7–12.

Navy Medicine, *Instructor Requirements for Navy Medicine Training Support Center*, Falls Church, Va.: U.S. Navy, Bureau of Medicine and Surgery, 2018. As of May 24, 2018:
https://www.med.navy.mil/sites/nmtsc/sitepages/instreq.html

Navy Personnel Command, *HM NEC Manning Snapshot April 2018*, Millington, Tenn.: U.S. Navy, 2018. As of August 9, 2018:
https://www.public.navy.mil/bupers-npc/enlisted/detailing/medical/Pages/default2.aspx

Navy Recruiting Command, *Medical Support Careers*, Millington, Tenn., 2018. As of May 24, 2018:
https://www.navy.com/careers/medical-support

Nelson, Karen, Maria Pitaro, Andrew Tzellas, and Audrey Lum, "Practice Profile. Transforming the Role of Medical Assistants in Chronic Disease Management," *Health Affairs*, Vol. 29, No. 5, May 2010, pp. 963–965.

Nielson, Matthew K., *Revolutionizing Mental Health Care Delivery in the United States Air Force by Shifting the Access Point to Primary Care*, unpublished doctoral dissertation, Maxwell Air Force Base, Ala.: Air Command and Staff College, Air University, 2016.

Pennsylvania Psychological Association, *PA Continuing Education Credit Requirements for Psychologists– Frequently Asked Questions*, Harrisburg, Pa., 2018. As of May 31, 2018:
https://cdn.ymaws.com/www.papsy.org/resource/resmgr/docs/CE_FAQs_for_web.pdf

Peterson, Alan L., Monty T. Baker, and Kelly R. McCarthy, "Combat Stress Casualties in Iraq. Part 1: Behavioral Health Consultation at an Expeditionary Medical Group," *Perspectives in Psychiatric Care*, Vol. 44, No. 3, 2008, pp. 146–158.

Potter, Aron, Monty Baker, Carmen Sanders, and Alan Peterson, "Combat Stress Reactions During Military Deployments: Evaluation of the Effectiveness of Combat Stress Control Treatment," *Journal of Mental Health Counseling*, Vol. 31, No. 2, 2009, pp. 137–148.

Public Law 114-328, National Defense Authorization Act for Fiscal Year 2017, 130 Stat 2000, 2016.

Puente, Antonio E., Russell Adams, William B. Barr, Shane S. Bush, Ronald M. Ruff, Jeffrey T. Barth, Donna Broshek, Sandra P. Koffler, Cecil Reynolds, Cheryl H. Silver, and Alexander I. Tröster, "The Use, Education, Training and Supervision of Neuropsychological Test Technicians (Psychometrists) in Clinical Practice. Official Statement of the National Academy of Neuropsychology," *Archives of Clinical Neuropsychology*, Vol. 21, No. 8, 2006, pp. 837–839.

Rapley, James, John Chin, Brian McCue, and Mathew Rariden, "Embedded Mental Health: Promotion of Psychological Hygiene Within a Submarine Squadron," *Military Medicine*, Vol. 182, No. 7, 2017, pp. e1675–e1680.

Robertson, Ivan T., and Mike Smith, "Personnel Selection," *Journal of Occupational and Organizational Psychology*, Vol. 74, No. 4, 2001, pp. 441–472. As of January 2, 2019:
https://onlinelibrary.wiley.com/doi/pdf/10.1348/096317901167479

Russell, Dale W., Ronald J. Whalen, Lyndon A. Riviere, Kristina Clarke-Walper, Paul D. Bliese, Darc D. Keller, Susan I. Pangelian, and Jeffrey L. Thomas, "Embedded Behavioral Health Providers: An Assessment with the Army National Guard," *Psychological Services*, Vol. 11, No. 3, 2014, p. 265.

Schendel, Christina, *Helping Your Patients Understand the Types of Military Mental Health Providers*, blog post, Falls Church, Va.: Psychological Health Center of Excellence, 2018. As of May 24, 2018:
http://pdhealth.mil/news/blog/helping-your-patients-understand-types-military-mental-health-providers

Smith-Forbes, Enrique, Cecilia Najera, and Donald Hawkins, "Combat Operational Stress Control in Iraq and Afghanistan: Army Occupational Therapy," *Military Medicine*, Vol. 179, No. 3, 2014, pp. 279–284.

Srinivasan, Jayakanth, and Julia DiBenigno, *Site Alpha Behavioral Health System of Care*, Massachusetts Institute of Technology, 2016. As of June 14, 2018:
https://dspace.mit.edu/bitstream/handle/1721.1/102556/Srinivasan%26DiBenigno2014SiteAlphaCurrentState Report.pdf?sequence=1

U.S. Air Force, *Mental Health Service*, Washington, D.C., 2017.

———, *Enlisted Mental Health Service*, Washington, D.C., 2018. As of June 4, 2018:
https://www.airforce.com/careers/detail/mental-health-service

U.S. Army, *Mental Health Specialist (68X)*, Washington, D.C., 2013a. As of May 24, 2018:
https://www.goarmy.com/reserve/jobs/browse/medical-and-emergency/mental-health-specialist.html

———, *Ready and Resilient Campaign: Embedded Behavioral Health*, Washington, D.C., 2013b. As of May 24, 2018:
https://www.army.mil/standto/archive_2013-08-13

———, *CMF 68 Smartbook*, Washington, D.C., 2017a.

———, *What Is the ASVAB Test?* fact sheet, Washington, D.C., 2017b. As of May 24, 2018:
https://www.goarmy.com/learn/understanding-the-asvab.html

U.S. Department of Defense, *Report of the Eleventh Quadrennial Review of Military Compensation, Supporting Research Papers*, Washington, D.C., 2012.

U.S. Department of Defense Task Force on Mental Health, *An Achievable Vision: Report of the Department of Defense Task Force on Mental Health*, Falls Church, Va.: Defense Health Board, 2007.

U.S. Department of the Air Force, *AFSC 4C0X1 Mental Health Service Specialty Career Field Education and Training Plan*, Washington, D.C., 2015.

U.S. Department of the Navy, *Catalog of Navy Training Courses (CANTRAC)*, Vol. II, Pensacola, Fla.: U.S. Naval Education and Training Command, undated, log-in required. As of June 26, 2018:
https://www.public.navy.mil/netc/Development.aspx

———, *BUMED Instruction 1510.23D, Hospital Corpsman Skills Basic*, Falls Church, Va.: Bureau of Medicine and Surgery, 2015. As of May 24, 2018:
http://www.med.navy.mil/directives/ExternalDirectives/1510.23D.pdf

———, *BUMED Instruction 1510.27 Hospital Corpsman Personnel Qualification Standards Program*, Falls Church, Va.: Bureau of Medicine and Surgery, 2017.

———, *MILPERSMAN 1910-120 Separation by Reason or Convenience of the Government—Physical or Mental Conditions*, Millington, Tenn.: Navy Personnel Command, 2012, now cancelled.

———, *Job Duty Task Analysis NEC 8485 Mental Health Technician*, fact sheet, Washington, D.C., 2013.

———, "Chapter 12, Education and Training," in U.S. Navy, *Manual of the Medical Department*, Change 158, Falls Church, Va.: U.S. Navy Bureau of Medicine and Surgery, November 1, 2016. As of May 24, 2018:
http://www.med.navy.mil/directives/Pub/MANMED%20CHANGE%20158.pdf

Weathers, Frank W., Brett T. Litz, Terence M. Keane, Patrick A. Palmieri, Brian P. Marx, and Paula P. Schnurr, *The PTSD Checklist for DSM-5 (PCL-5)*, diagnostic instrument, National Center for PTSD, 2013. As of August 10, 2018:
https://www.ptsd.va.gov/professional/assessment/adult-sr/ptsd-checklist.asp

Wechsler, David, *Wechsler Adult Intelligence Scale* (4th ed.), San Antonio, Tex.: Psychological Corporation, 2008.

West Virginia Board of Examiners of Psychologists, *Guidelines for Continuing Education*, Charleston, W. Va., 2018. As of May 31, 2018:
https://psychbd.wv.gov/cont-ed/Documents/CE%20Guidelines.pdf

What Are the 12 Core Functions of a Drug and Alcohol Counselor? blog post, Mokena, Ill.: Family First Intervention, 2018. As of May 24, 2018:
https://family-intervention.com/blog/12-core-functions-drug-alcohol-counselor/

Will, Kristen K., Adriane I. Budavari, James A. Wilkens, Kenneth Mishark, and Zachary C. Hartsell, "A Hospitalist Postgraduate Training Program for Physician Assistants," *Journal of Hospital Medicine*, Vol. 5, No. 2, February 2010, pp. 94–98.